THE SUNDAY TIMES
ABC
DIET AND BODYPLAN

The Eight-Week Course That Can
Re-shape Your Life

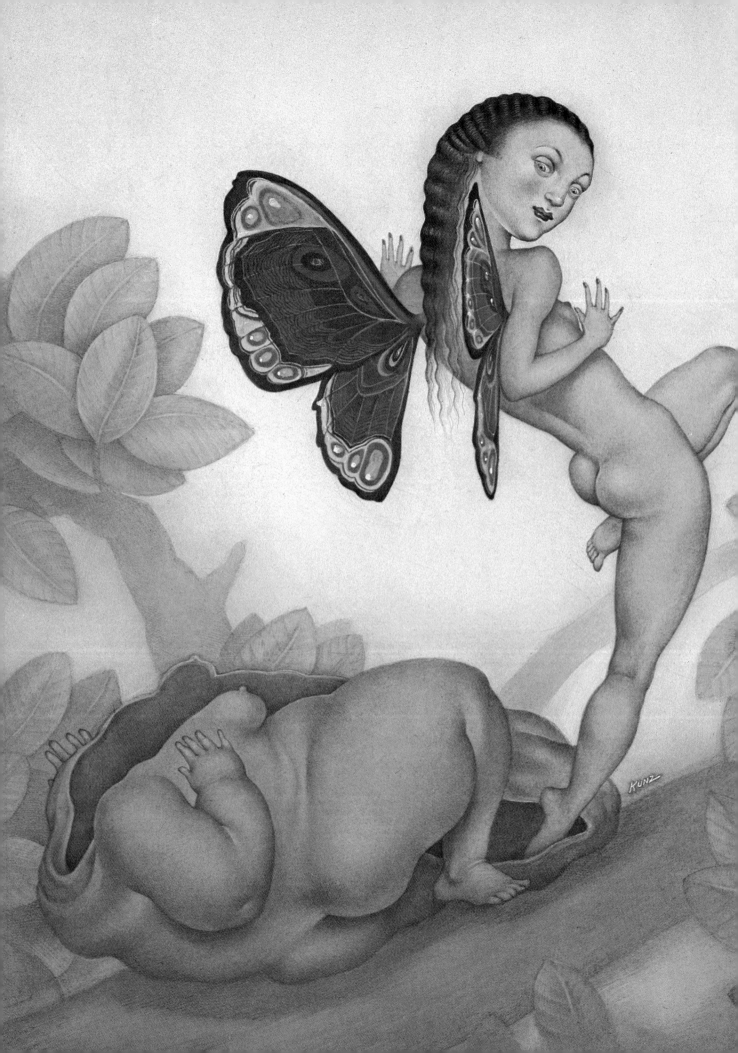

THE SUNDAY TIMES
ABC
DIET AND BODYPLAN

The Eight-Week Course That Can Re-shape Your Life

Oliver Gillie and Susana Raby

Recipes by
Dinah Morrison

Hutchinson
London Melbourne Sydney Auckland Johannesburg

Hutchinson & Co (Publishers) Ltd

An imprint of the Hutchinson Publishing Group
17-21 Conway Street, London W1P 6JD

Hutchinson Group (Australia) Pty Ltd
PO Box 496, 16-22 Church Street, Hawthorne, Melbourne, Victoria 3122
PO Box 151, Broadway, New South Wales 277

Hutchinson Group (NZ) Ltd
32-34 View Road, PO Box 40-086, Glenfield, Auckland 10

Hutchinson Group (SA) Pty Ltd
PO Box 337, Bergvlei 2012, South Africa

First published in The Sunday Times Magazine in April-June 1984

This expanded edition first published in July 1984

© Oliver Gillie, Susana Raby and The Sunday Times, 1984

Edited, designed and produced by Michael Balfour Ltd
3 Wedgwood Mews, Greek Street, London W1V 5LW

Project co-ordinator   Michael Balfour
Exercise consultant   Esme Newton-Dunn
Artwork and photography   Credits on page 144
Additional picture research   Sue Bolsom Morris
Designers   Field Wylie & Company
Production Consultant   Dee Maple
Typesetting   H & J Graphics Ltd
Reproduction   Bridge Graphics Ltd
Printing and binding   Severn Valley Press Ltd

British Library Cataloguing in Publication Data

Gillie, Oliver
  The Sunday Times ABC Diet and Bodyplan
  1. Reducing
  1. Title   11. Raby,   Susana
  613.2'5   RM222.2

ISBN 0 09 158911 8

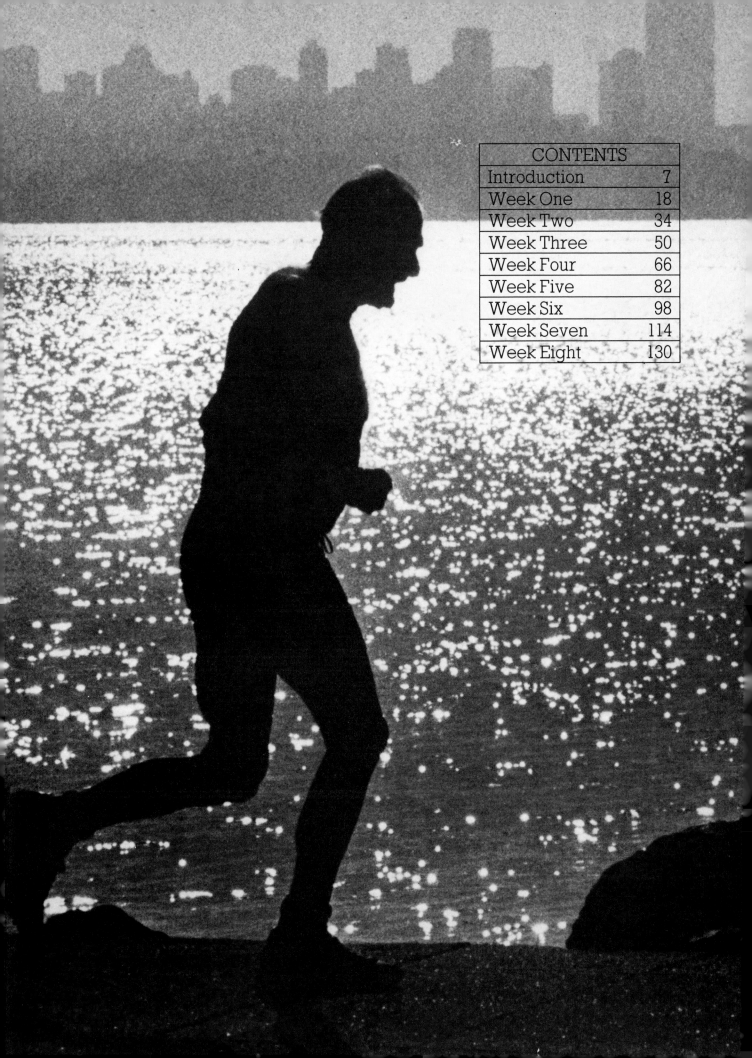

CONTENTS

Acknowledgements

We would like to thank the many people who have helped to make this book possible. In particular we would like to thank Professor John Durnin for his advice about exercise and for reading sections of the book, and Dr David Jenkins and Dr Hellmut Otto, whose research into food and physiology has made it possible for us to devise the Constant Energy Diet. Gilvrie Misstear deserves special thanks for the hard work and imagination she brought to the job of art director of *The Sunday Times Magazine* series on which this book is based. We are also indebted to Brenda Jones for the effort and careful thought she brought to bear on our manuscript, and to Geoffrey Cannon for friendly help.

We are grateful to Norman Harris, director of *The Sunday Times Fun Run*, and Cliff Temple for their help and advice about running, John Lovesey for his advice about swimming training, and Esme Newton-Dunn for her advice about exercises. We thank Dr Eric Newsholme for his advice on the effects of exercise on metabolism. We are grateful to Dr William Hartston for bringing his expertise in psychology to bear in composing our slimmer's quiz. Dr Glenn Wilson of the Institute of Psychiatry, London, and Professor David Denison of the Brompton Hospital, London, deserve our special thanks for their cooperation in research projects based on the ABC Diet and Bodyplan. Lastly, we would like to thank Michael Balfour for the skilful guidance which made it possible to produce this book in such good time.

Oliver Gillie
Susana Raby

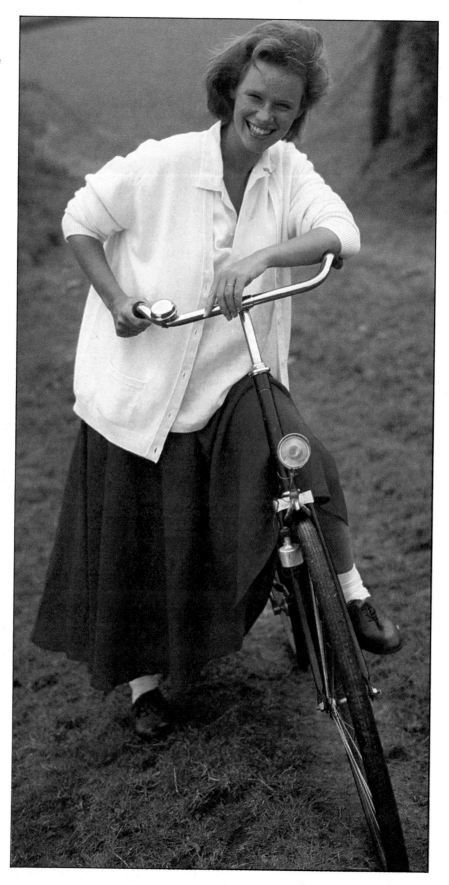

INTRODUCTION

The ABC Diet and Bodyplan is a comprehensive plan for losing weight, getting fit and establishing a healthy lifestyle. It will help you to look good because the diet promotes health and the exercise promotes fitness and improves body shape. Our exercise programme is carefully graduated so that even those who have not taken exercise for several years can start, and build up steadily, while for those who want to do more, it leads in easy stages to jogging and running.

But the ABC Diet and Bodyplan is not just another exercise programme – it includes the Constant Energy Diet. There is nothing faddy about this diet. You will not be asked, as on some diets, to forsake delicious food in favour of a lot of meat and little else or worthy but boring baked beans and bran. You can throw away the calorie charts and the bathroom scales – you won't need them with the Constant Energy Diet.

A lot has been written about the dangers of being overweight, but the fact is that a moderate excess of weight is probably not as much as a hazard as many of the diets undertaken to correct it. In order to promote health, slimming must be carried out in the right way. High-fat diets, for instance, increase the risk of heart disease. The Constant Energy Diet is completely safe and incorporates the latest medical advice for avoiding heart disease.

The Constant Energy Diet is based on the latest scientific findings showing how a steady level of sugar can be maintained in the blood so as to avoid hunger and fatigue. It introduces some precision into a subject which, hitherto, has been guesswork. Nevertheless it is beautifully simple to follow. We believe that it provides the commonsense approach that so many dieters are looking for.

The ABC Bodyplan takes into account another vital link in achieving a healthy lifestyle: behaviour. By behaviour we mean the patterns which shape our lives, from feelings that drive us to overeat to the way we actually eat what's on our plate; from the way we deal with other people to the

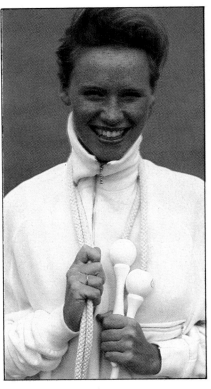

way we think of our bodies; from the way we react to stress and failure to the messages we constantly give ourselves, whether we realize it or not.

You may eat normally most of the time but go on binges that leave you feeling guilty and fat. You may eat sensibly but simply eat too much. You may eat in reasonable quantities but eat the wrong foods. You may drink too much. Potent psychological factors are involved in all these problems. The ABC Bodyplan will show you how you can identify these problems and how they can be corrected.

Some people who eat very little are overweight because they take so little exercise – and exercise is especially important for those people whom we might call professional dieters. They are the people who have slowed their metabolism down so much by constant dieting that, despite eating very little, their weight stays at the same level. And their diet provides so few nutrients that their health may be compromised. Exercise breaks this cycle.

The person who was once very active and fit but is now overweight and plays games only

once a week can also benefit from the ABC Bodyplan, which will show such people what they can do to become slim and super-fit again. The Constant Energy Diet is first-class for games players and athletes because it provides a steady energy supply over a long period, enhancing stamina and competitiveness.

The basic aim of the ABC Bodyplan is to help you shape up by developing muscle and shedding fat in easy stages, and to establish healthy patterns of exercise and eating which you can continue indefinitely. It also shows you how to control stress, which may be causing you to overeat. It helps break the cycle of unduly high expectations, failure and guilt which plague habitual dieters, it guides you through the patches when morale or motivation are low, and shows you how to harness the power of your imagination to achieve your goals.

The health pay-off

People who are overweight have a substantially increased risk of dying suddenly from a heart attack or stroke. They also have an increased risk of suffering from heart disease, high blood pressure, diabetes, gallbladder disease, arthritis and certain types of cancer. Health can be improved and these hazards reduced by reducing weight, but many people who have been overweight in the past still seem to carry an above-average risk of suffering from these diseases. One reason for this is that when they slim on low-carbohydrate diets, which by definition contain a high proportion of fat, they perpetuate the abnormal body chemistry which is associated with an increased risk of disease. The Constant Energy Diet avoids this problem, following as it does the recommendations of the reports on heart disease, dietary fibre and obesity of the Royal College of Physicians as well as the recommendations of the US Senate Committee on Nutrition.

Many studies have shown that active people in their 50s and 60s can have heart and lung functions as good as or better than an unfit 20 year old. But exercise does even more to preserve a youthful body.

It is vital for conserving muscles and bones. Astronauts lose calcium from their bones because they cannot exercise in space. The same thing happens progressively to men and women as they take less exercise with increasing age. Exercise helps to prevent loss of calcium because the stresses on bone resulting from exercise cause active reinforcement; exercise also helps to maintain the flexibility of joints and prevent arthritis. Use it or lose it, as the exercise experts say.

However, the most immediate benefit of exercise is definitely psychological. Exercise is a natural tranquillizer – it makes people better able to handle both physical and emotional stress. It can also relieve deep depression, increase self-confidence and reduce feelings of hostility and anger as well as causing a very pleasant feeling of euphoria – the exercise high.

How Much Weight Will You Lose?

The ABC Diet and Bodyplan aims at promoting fat loss and the effect of this for most people is loss of weight as well as improvement in shape. Many people will lose a steady one or two pounds a week on the ABC Bodyplan.

Obession with body weight, however, may prevent you from getting the most out of the ABC Bodyplan and we suggest that you do not weigh yourself more than once a week at most. In fact it is better not to weigh yourself at all, but to monitor your fat loss with a tape measure.

Loss of weight begins slowly on the ABC Bodyplan. Do not expect to lose much more than a pound, if that, in the first week. As you get fitter you will be able to take more exercise, and at the same time you will get going with the diet and behaviour programme and so lose weight more quickly.

With other types of diet it is common to lose several pounds in the first week – but this loss is highly deceptive. It occurs because the glycogen (starch) stores in the liver are depleted rapidly at the start of the diet and a

lot of water is released from the body. After the first few weeks weight loss on these diets is much slower – about one or two pounds a week – yet the price is a perpetual feeling of semi-starvation. At the end of the diet the body rebuilds its glycogen in the liver and several pounds of weight immediately go back on as consumption is allowed to return to normal.

The ABC Bodyplan is based on proven methods of weight loss, so it is possible to predict from published scientific work the weight loss which might be expected. We have also tested the plan on volunteers, whose good results confirmed the merits of the method. How much weight you lose will depend how closely you are able to follow the three sections (the A, B and C) of the programme. But even if you follow only one section you can expect to get slimmer.

Exercise alone has been found in a number of studies to produce weight loss of up to two pounds a week, and average losses of half a stone in about three months. As much as a stone may be lost in just two months through exercise alone. *The Sunday Times* 'Getting in Shape' programme was organized by Geoffrey Cannon and assessed by Professor David Denison of the Institute of Cardiology at the Brompton Hospital, London. Men lost an average of 5lbs, and women an average of 3lbs, over eight months on an aerobic exercise programme, when they weren't even aiming to lose weight, only to get fit. Some people lost up to a stone.

Programmes aimed at changing the *way* you eat (as opposed to *what* you eat) have been shown to result in average losses of a pound a week at first and 10 pounds in a year. Slimmers who involve their family in such behaviour modification programmes are likely to be twice as successful, and weight losses of two pounds a week are possible with this method alone.

It is more difficult to predict how much weight may be lost on the Constant Energy Diet because it involves new ideas. However, it

builds on the old idea of a more natural diet with less sugar, less fat and more fibre. Depending very much on individuals and the type of food they ate previously, the Constant Energy Diet might be expected to lead to a weight loss of up to three pounds a week – over a stone and a half in eight weeks – for some people. Most people will probably progress at a rate of a pound a week but find that they can happily continue with our programme for months and so still lose a stone in weight eventually. Others may not lose much weight but will still notice an improvement in their shape.

Results of the ABC Diet and Bodyplan

Although the ABC Diet and Bodyplan is not aiming exclusively at weight loss, it has produced better results than diets the specific aim of which is weight loss. Most of these diets, which restrict calorie intake, produce weight loss for only one in five people who start on them, and are only really successful for about one person in 200. This is because so many people give up restrictive diets when they can no longer stand the hunger and the boring food. More than half our volunteers lost some weight and one person in five lost 10-14 lbs in eight weeks; most had tried other diets before but with much less success. Those who did not lose weight were still pleased with the programme, and several noticed a loss of fat.

All those who undertook the ABC Bodyplan remarked that they felt better. Greater energy, a general sense of well-being, and sounder, more refreshing sleep were among the most commonly reported benefits. Hunger was not a problem. Several said that they enjoyed their food more and felt less guilty about eating. The few who lost no weight still appreciated the ABC Bodyplan because they were able to stop worrying about calories and the quantity of food they ate; they were enjoying their food yet not putting on weight. Valuable psychological effects included looking better, feeling calmer, increased confidence, and greater assertiveness in making decisions and choices.

Why Exercise?

Maybe you only have a few pounds to lose. You find most exercises difficult and boring. Do you really need to punish yourself with exercise when you can starve for a week and watch the weight fall off?

Or perhaps you are two or three stone overweight and wouldn't dream of being seen in a track suit until you have lost at least a stone. It might seem logical to diet for a week or two before you start running.

But, however much you need to lose, the answer is clearcut: proper exercise not only helps you shed fat more easily than cranky diets but is also crucial to staying slim – and the fatter you are, the sooner you will see results.

It was once believed that cutting calorie intake was the only way to lose weight, that you would have to walk 32 miles to lose a pound, and that exercise only sharpened your appetite. But recent research shows that exercise sets up various changes in your body which help you to slim, and as former fatties Geoffrey Cannon ('Dieting Makes You Fat') and Mary Ellen Pinkham ('Mary Ellen's Help Yourself Diet') attest, it can help you stay slim without starving yourself.

At first you may have to watch your food intake too, but calorie counting is no substitute for regular, vigorous exercise. Once you start exercising you will soon be able to eat enough food to nourish and satisfy yourself and still lose weight.

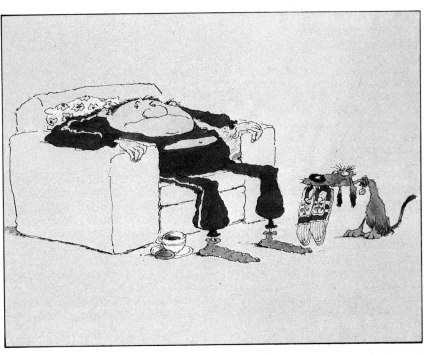

PHYSICS IS HELPING YOU

There is one encouraging fact for everyone who is overweight. The heavier you are the faster you lose weight when you take exercise. There is no way you can be cheated of the benefits of this law of physics: the heavier you are the more work you do in any standard exercise and therefore the more energy and fat you burn up. All you have to do is begin exercising and you begin winning. This is not just a theory. The heavier people have been found to lose weight fastest in exercise programmes.

Exercise actually reduces hunger

In people who take little exercise, appetite signals seem to go astray, so that you feel hunger inappropriately. Exercise actually improves the efficiency of the appetite regulation centre in your brain so that you feel hunger only when you *need* food. A complex series of hormonal changes occurs so that your body can distinguish between real hunger and false appetite. This is what happens when you exercise:

1. You'll burn calories faster

Exercise boosts the body's basal metabolic rate (BMR: the rate at which you burn up calories) by up to 30 per cent, according to research by the late Dr Lars Hermansen of the Institute of Work Physiology in Oslo. Even after 24 hours it is still raised by almost 10 per cent. With regular exercise your BMR may be raised permanently by as much as 15 per cent, so that you use more energy not only while you exercise but all the time, even while you sleep. This means that if you take more exercise you will steadily lose fat or be able to eat considerably more food without putting on weight.

2. You'll be firing on all cylinders

As your exercise routine continues and fat is replaced by more active muscle, your body will produce more heat, because your metabolism is boosted indirectly by the higher 'idling speed' of your active body, as well as directly by the exercise you take each day. Muscle tissue burns more calories than fat – so the more muscle you have the more food calories you are able to burn.

3. Your weight will stabilize at a lower point

Many scientists now believe that exercise lowers the 'set point', the point at which your weight tends to stabilize. Exercise is the only way of lowering this set point permanently. Without exercise, attempts to slim demand enormous self-control and are likely to become increasingly difficult because body weight tends to return automatically to the set point. Strong-willed individuals who have endured the pangs of dieting may end up weighing less, but much of the loss will have been muscle. When muscle is lost by dieting the ability to burn up energy from food decreases and so less food must be eaten if weight is not to be put on more quickly than before.

Furthermore, with restrictive dieting the metabolic rate of the body drops because the body, designed for survival, under-standably interprets lack of food

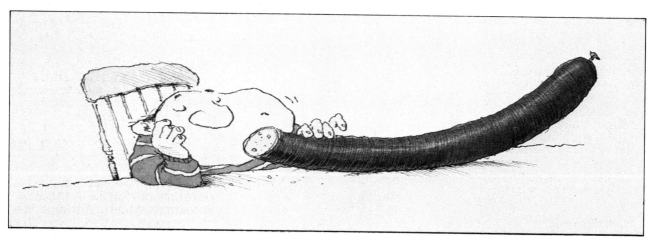

as a crisis that requires it to conserve energy by ticking over more slowly. To get slimmer by dieting with little or no exercise, it is necessary to keep on reducing the intake of calories.

4. You will be more shapely

Those who do continue to diet successfully by self-starvation often acquire a rather drawn appearance, with thin sagging skin supported by insufficient muscle.

The same loss of muscle occurs after years of a sedentary lifestyle, and to most people as they get older and take less exercise. The figure then begins to sag even though body weight may change hardly at all. Exercise produces a better body shape and a more youthful appearance. Fat particularly tends to go from the hips with walking or running. Even if your weight changes only a little the exercise in our programme will change your shape for the better.

5. More exercise and more nutrients

Without exercise health suffers because it is impossible to balance the diet properly. A diet adequate in nutrients contains too many calories for someone who is inactive and so weight is gained. Alternatively, if the diet contains only the small number of calories necessary for a sedentary life then it is inadequate in nutrients and so health may suffer. Balancing the energy and nutrient content of the diet can be a problem at any age but it is particularly difficult for older people who have become accustomed to leading very inactive lives. The ABC Bodyplan

is graduated so that almost anybody, from amateur sports enthusiasts to the old or unfit, can find a level that suits them.

How the Constant Energy Diet Works

If the word diet conjures up thoughts of starvation then you will be pleasantly surprised by the Constant Energy Diet. Its aim of satisfying hunger and providing ample energy all day long makes it different from other slimming diets. It is based on a new understanding of the way in which food is absorbed by the body and either converted into energy or stored as fat. This is of importance not only to slimmers but also to athletes and anyone who regularly suffers from the sort of tiredness which is relieved by nibbling a biscuit or sucking a sweet.

Unlike other slimming regimes, the Constant Energy Diet does not aim to starve slimmers in the hope of creating an energy gap which, if it can be sustained, leads to loss of weight. By reducing hunger to a minimum it reduces the body's own stimulus to overeat, and in this way the intake of surplus energy can be cut down with minimum effort, resulting in loss of fat. The Constant Energy Diet also aims to alter the body chemistry so that it ceases to favour fat storage.

Our diet helps to limit both hunger and unwanted fat storage in the body by discouraging foods which overload the body with sugar and fat, and by favouring carbohydrate foods which release

their sugar slowly. As a result insulin – the hormone in the body which is important in controlling use of energy, storage of fat and probably hunger itself – is kept at a more regular level.

At the same time our exercise programme helps to sensitize the muscles to insulin. The combined effect of these two measures is to change the way the body uses energy. Wild fluctuations in blood sugar which may lead to the storage of fat are much less likely to occur, and the feeling of tiredness which follows when blood sugar is low should occur less frequently. The ABC Diet and Bodyplan thus aims to break the addictive cycle of fatigue, hunger and overeating which inevitably leads to weight gain.

Many people who are overweight eat too much fat and sugar. Such a diet, combined with too little exercise, seems to throw the body into a chemical state resembling starvation – even though the person may actually be eating more food than the body needs. Lack of exercise makes the muscles insensitive to insulin so

---

THE CONSTANT ENERGY DIET

The Constant Energy Diet is based on these principles:
- Less use of sugar.
- Use of fat in careful combination with starchy foods.
- Omission of high fat foods.
- Increased proportion of wholefoods (not just wholemeal foods).
- Increased bulk from vegetables and fruit.

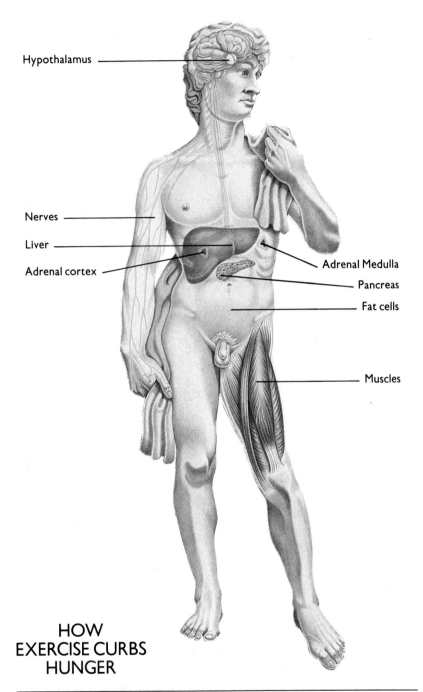

HOW
EXERCISE CURBS
HUNGER

that much of the sugar (in the form of glucose) accumulates in the blood and there may be a delay before it is stored. At the same time large quantities of fat in the blood further slow down the use of sugar by body tissues, causing what is known as insulin resistance.

There are two ways in which this insulin resistance can be reversed, says Dr M.G. Clark, nutrition expert at the Australian Government's Human Nutrition Research Institute in Adelaide, in a major review of the subject in 'The Lancet' (November 1983): by changing to a diet low in fat and high in carbohydrates other than sugar and by physical training. Clark points out that several studies in animals and man show that physical training increases uptake of sugar by muscle so that more energy is used; insulin and sugar levels in the blood then return to normal. As a result body fat can be more easily broken down and excess weight can begin to be shed more easily. This is what the ABC Diet and Bodyplan aims to do.

Starting the ABC Diet and Bodyplan

Our Bodyplan is carefully designed to change your diet and your lifestyle in a series of easy stages. We start off with a preliminary week when we ask you to do four things:
1. Test yourself with the ABC Body Quiz which follows to find out what your special problems are.
2. Keep your ABC Diary, noting every item of food and drink you consume in one week.
3. Work out which is the best exercise for you and begin now by walking for up to half an hour every other day, if you can.
4. At the end of the week take the ABC Road Test and select the right type of exercise for your age and level of fitness.
In the following week, Week One, you start to make changes in your diet, begin a planned exercise programme and start to analyze any eating problems.

How exercise curbs hunger: *Vigorous exercise, far from sharpening appetite, actually blunts it. It tunes up the appetite control centre in the brain so that it becomes more sensitive to chemical changes in the body which indicate when enough food has been eaten.* **The liver** *is prompted by exercise to increase the release of stored glucose. As glucose levels in blood and brain rise, the hypothalamus, which governs appetite, switches off feelings of hunger.* **The hypothalamus** *is tuned up by exercise. Unless you walk three miles a day or do the equivalent exercise, the hypothalamus prepares for starvation or hibernation – it makes body functions slow down and increases appetite. Following exercise,* **the nerves** *produce more of two anti-hunger chemicals – serotonin, which reduces cravings for carbohydrate, and dopamine, which curbs appetite because of its stimulant properties.* **The adrenal medulla** *(inner part of the adrenal glands) is stimulated to increase its output of the hormones adrenalin and noradrenalin. Both are stimulants which curtail hunger by mobilizing fat, drawing it out of fat cells into the blood. This acts as a signal of fullness. With exercise* **the adrenal cortex** *(outer part of the adrenal gland) produces less of the hormone cortisol, which promotes hunger and the storage of fat.* **Fat cells** *are prompted by exercise to release glycerol and fats into the blood, curbing hunger.* **The pancreas** *receives signals from the hypothalamus to secrete less hunger-inducing insulin. Regular exercise speeds up insulin transfer from blood to spinal fluid and brain.* **Muscles** *become more sensitive as a result of exercise; insulin production and hunger pangs are switched off sooner.*

1. The ABC Body Quiz

Few of us have completely regular or predictable patterns of eating or taking exercise. In the following tale of a reasonably eventful Friday and Saturday, choose those of the statements which you think, on balance, are true of you. There is no restriction to the number of statements with which you choose to agree. Do not feel obliged to try to choose one in preference to another; just answer honestly, putting a ring round the index number of each statement which you think most accurately describes you and your attitudes.

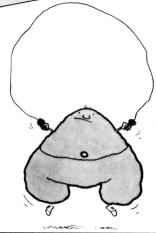

It's a beautiful Friday morning; time for breakfast:

1a I often skip not only breakfast but lunch too.
1b I'd rather stay in bed a bit longer and miss breakfast.
1c A full English breakfast sets me up for the day, even if I know I'll be having lunch and dinner too.
1d I take sugar in my tea or coffee.
1e I just grab anything to eat; there's always food around at home.
1f My choice would be a croissant with butter and cherry jam and freshly ground coffee.
1g The more spare time I have for breakfast, the more I eat.

Off to work, or settling down to work; time for a break:

2a I can't resist a biscuit when it's offered with tea or coffee.
2b I'm often tempted by a sausage roll, doughnut or pastry.
2c I tend to eat more when I feel there's not much work to do.
2d I tend to eat more when I feel there's too much work to do.

Lunchtime: someone important has retired and there's a sumptuous buffet in his honour:

3a I lose count of how much I'm drinking when my glass is constantly topped up.
3b When the spread is well prepared and varied, I like to try a bit of everything if I can.
3c If there's nobody I know at the party, I'll eat more out of sheer boredom.
3d I'll plump for some salmon mousse and asparagus with hollandaise sauce.
3e I'm quite capable of stuffing myself on buffet nosh, then not eating properly for days after.
3f I'm liable to eat more if I'm annoyed after a bad morning.
3g It makes a change from my usual lunch of something and chips.

Work is over for the day, and it's time to relax:

4a I'm quite likely to join some friends for a drink in the pub.
4b If I do go out for a drink, I'll probably have nuts or crisps too.

The party, still sober, dissolves into smaller groups:

5a I'll often be one of those who head for a fish and chip shop, hamburger joint or other convenient take-away.

Friday night or Saturday morning is time for a trip round the supermarket, gathering in goodies for the weekend:

6a I usually throw some sweets or chocolate into the basket.
6b I always make sure that the larder will be well stocked.
6c I like to keep a supply of nuts or biscuits in case I fancy a little snack at any time.
6d I prefer to go to several specialist shops.
6e I go to the shop nearest home, even though it's more expensive and the selection isn't so good.

At last some free time at home:

7a I sometimes find myself prowling about, looking for I know not what, then end up in the kitchen eating something.
7b I find it hard to walk past a food-laden table or tray without sampling some.
7c At mealtimes, I'm liable to eat up the bits other members of the family leave on their plates.
7d I find cooking relaxing, so I'll prepare a good meal and maybe invite some friends over to share it.
7e It's hard to get out of a comfortable chair, even when dinner beckons.
7f The busier I am, the less I eat.

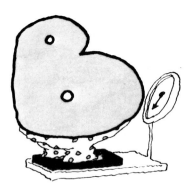

An old friend phones out of the blue and you're delighted to have the chance to meet up again:

8a A cream tea would be a nice idea.

He can't make it for tea anyway, so you agree to meet at his flat then to go out for dinner. The flat is on the second floor:

9a I'd take the lift rather than walk up.
9b I hope he offers me a drink before we set off for the meal.

You approach the task of selecting a restaurant. Among your important criteria, you'd like a restaurant which

10a is not mean with its portions.
10b is near tube, bus or parking space, so there won't be far to walk.
10c is licensed
10d has a relaxed atmosphere which will help you eat away the day's worries.
10e you know has a good chef and is likely to include an exotic dish on its menu.

When choosing what to eat:

11a I may not have eaten all day, so I could eat what I please.
11b I'd consider ordering an extra dish from a tempting menu, just to try a new taste.
11c I go for dishes with a delicate flavour that won't detract from the fine wine.
11d An aperitif before, and wine or beer with the meal, help the food down.
11e I can never resist the savoury nibbles on the tables while I'm waiting for the order to arrive.
11f When the sweet trolley comes round, I can always find room for something.
11g I'll happily gnaw my way through a chunk of cheese rather than having a pudding.

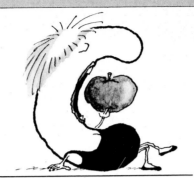

During the meal:

12a If my companion overeats, I tend to do so too.
12b I like to sample food from my companion's choices.
12c I tend to eat more if the mood is not relaxed.
12d To see me picking at food in a restaurant, nobody would guess how much I eat when I'm alone.
12e I'd rather have a side salad with a tasty dressing than a plain selection of vegetables.

After the meal:

13a I like to go away with a sweet taste in my mouth.
13b I'll maybe have a liqueur, or just another drink, to round off the evening.
13c I sometimes feel pangs of guilt when I realise how much I've eaten.
13d I might have a dessert wine such as a Sauternes or a Barsac, or perhaps a glass of Armagnac.
13e I'd get a bus or taxi home, rather than take a 15-minute walk.

All in all, it's been a pretty average couple of days, with an average food intake. On an average day:

14a I have at least one glass of wine or spirits or half a pint of beer or cider.
14b I have a canned soft drink.
14c I may munch something between meals, just to pass the time.
14d I don't have average days – my eating habits are far too chaotic.
14e I don't play any sport; in fact I don't even in an average week.

Food can have a number of different effects on me, besides satisfying my hunger:

15a When I'm tired, eating something sweet can give me energy.
15b When I'm troubled, eating something has a soothing effect.
15c When there's nothing to do, eating is a way of passing the time.

All these questions! It's enough to give you an appetite:

16a I like to eat when I'm lonely, frustrated or anxious.
16b I like to eat when I'm bored, or at a loose end.
16c I can eat sweets at any time.
16d I often take too large a helping and feel I have to eat it.
16e I can easily stay away from food, but once I start eating, it can be hard to stop.

Now transfer all your ringed choices to the list of numbers below:

Binger	Lazy-bones	Guzzler	Sugar Sweetie	Nibbler	Gourmet	Monotonous Muncher	Fatty Feeder	Emotional Eater	Daily Drinker
1a	(1b)	1c	1d	1e	(1f)	(1g)	2b	2d	3a
3e	6e	(6b)	(6a)	(2a)	3d	2c	3g	(3f)	4a
11a	7e	(7c)	(11f)	3b	6d	3c	(4b)	(7a)	9b
12d	(9a)	(10a)	(13a)	6c	7d	(7f)	5a	(10d)	(10c)
(13c)	(10b)	11b	(14b)	(7b)	10e	(14c)	8a)	12c	11d
14d	(13e)	12a)	(15a)	(11e)	11c	(15c)	11g	(15b)	13b
16e	(14e)	(16d)	16c	12b	13d	(16b)	(12e)	(16a)	14a

The column which contains the highest number of your answers shows your over-eating style. Four or more items in *any* column should be seen as a danger sign, and an indication that you probably indulge too much in that behaviour. Your score may be high in more than one category. Don't be depressed if it is; it means you have definite habits which are the basis of your weight problems, and the ABC Diet and Bodyplan will help you change them.

Now we will examine your answers to the ABC Body Quiz in detail.

Binger
You are obsessed with food. When not on a strict diet, you feel guilty because of bingeing on forbidden goodies. Yet your problem is not so much food itself as your attitudes and how you eat. We deal with bingeing at length in Week One, but take the first step towards changing your eating style now. Plan three balanced meals for tomorrow and eat them whether or not you feel hungry.

Lazybones
You may not eat too much, but what you do eat turns into fat because you don't burn it off with exercise. Over the next few weeks, you can gradually build up to a regular programme of vigorous exercise (essential to losing fat and becoming more energetic) with the ABC Diet and Bodyplan. In the meantime start walking and make small changes: use stairs instead of lifts, walk to work or the shops instead of taking the car.

Guzzler
Your meals are relatively well balanced, but you eat too much: perhaps a hearty breakfast, followed by a business lunch and a large cooked meal at night. If so, start now to cut down on the non-essentials – snacks, starters, puddings and extra helpings. Later we'll offer more detailed hints to help you eat less and stay satisfied.

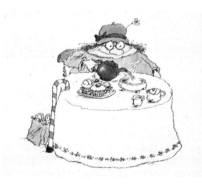

Sugar Sweetie
Too much sugar gives you highs and lows of energy and disrupts your body chemistry. If you overeat sugary foods, your energy peaks then drops drastically, leaving you craving yet more sugar. We will tell you how to alter your diet to introduce palatable foods which release energy slowly, and keep you satisfied longer, while you phase out sugar. Within a few weeks, foods you thought you couldn't do without will taste too sweet.

Nibbler
You eat in such a thoughtless, haphazard way that you can't remember what you ate or where and when you ate it. Almost anything – a chat, the sight of a baker's window or a bowl of peanuts – is the cue for food. To impose order you need to plan your eating (including snacks if you adjust meal sizes accordingly). Use the ABC Diary, which follows, to keep track of your intake.

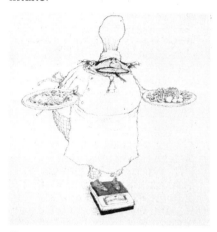

Gourmet
If your love of fine food is showing on your waistline, use your knowledge and discrimination to replace rich dishes with simple but delicious food that follows the guidelines of the Constant Energy Diet, which we introduce in Week One.

Monotonous Muncher
Boredom drives you to eat more than you want or need. Food will tempt you less often if you plan your time better; decide in advance how long you will read or watch television before switching to another activity, and plan exactly *when* you will have a drink or a snack. Following the three elements of the ABC Diet and Bodyplan will encourage you to structure your time to avoid boredom.

Fatty Feeder
Whether from ignorance or foolhardiness, perhaps from habits acquired in childhood, you are eating far too much fat, thereby jeopardizing your health as well as spreading your waistline. The Constant Energy Diet allows you to eat moderate amounts of fat, but will direct you to truly satisfying lower fat foods.

Emotional Eater
Worry, fear, tension and depression can cause you to eat too much or too often. The B for Behaviour sections each week will guide you to the best relaxation techniques, and the A for Activity sections will help you work off frustration or worry. Meanwhile, use your ABC Diary to note the people and situations that make you anxious and upset – and avoid them until you have cultivated more detachment.

Daily Drinker
Most alcoholic drinks are laden with sugar (and calories). Up to half a bottle of wine with a meal is fine, unless you're too fat already. More than half and your regular drinking could not only be making you fat but also might be hazardous to health. Later in the book we will be focusing on what to drink and how to drink to avoid extra calories.

2. How to keep your ABC Diary

Before you can change your lifestyle you need to keep a record of what you are doing at present, so that you can see how it should be changed. We provide you with an ABC Diary in which you should record daily your Activity or exercise, your eating Behaviour and your Consumption of food–see page 16.

Most people launch into diets without thinking much about the way their eating habits and behaviour may be causing them to overeat. For instance, it is helpful to know what triggers off feelings of hunger, how many times a day you eat, whether food makes you feel drowsy or more energetic or relieves tension, and how much exercise you take in an average day. By keeping the ABC Diary you will be able to work out the connections between all these factors in your life style and the food you eat. This is how to do it.

Begin with measurements

When you step on the scales for your ritual weigh-in, do you feel despondent if you are over the 'ideal' weight for your height and frame? Or proud if you weigh the same as you did as a super-fit 20-year old? Either way you could be wrong.

What the scales can't tell you is how much of your weight is muscle and how much is fat. Muscle is heavier than fat, so two people of the same height and age could weigh the same, yet one would be slim because he or she has a high proportion of muscle, and the other chubby because his or her weight is mainly fat.

The ABC Diet and Bodyplan aims at fat loss, not weight loss. After following it for a few weeks you should find that your shape improves even if your weight does not drop dramatically. You may even put on weight, but still lose inches of flab. This is how to find the flab:

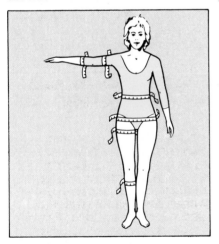

- Measure yourself at all the places shown in the diagram and make a note of them in your Diary. Check week by week how much trimmer you are getting.
- Men can take the belly test: breathe out and measure your waist at navel level with muscles relaxed. Breathe in and measure your chest at full expansion: if it is smaller than your waist, you are too fat.

Activity

In the activity column make a note of any regular exercise such as walking to work or shops, walking a dog, games, etc. Also make a special note of the walks you take in this preliminary week and the result of the ABC Road Test which follows.

Behaviour

This will be a crowded column referring to the other two. Each day keep track of the following and note the time of the day when they occur.

- How you feel when you wake up, eg: tired, refreshed, headach.
- How you feel after exercising, eg: tired, invigorated, more or less hungry than before.
- How hungry you feel. Any time you feel hungry rate your desire to eat on a scale from 1 to 5, whether you eat or not. Make the record *before* you eat. The point of this is to see if there is a pattern to your hunger. Eating is very much a matter of habit and is often triggered by situations or by stress rather than by real hunger.
- How you felt before eating, eg bored, lonely, edgy, frustrated, angry. This information is important because it will help to make you more sensitive to internal signals, which at present you may not differentiate from each other. Again, record these feelings in your diary before you eat.
- Any external cues which precede eating, eg: switching on the TV, the sight of a tea or coffee trolley at work, sitting down to tackle a particularly difficult problem, the arrival of friends. Note where you ate, eg: in the living room, in the kitchen, at the desk, in the street. Make a note of who was with you.
- How you feel after eating, Include physical feelings (eg: satisfied, too full, lethargic) and emotions (eg: relaxed, contented, guilty).

Consumption

Record everything you eat during the day, including all snacks and drinks, in the appropriate time slot. Don't wait too long, though. Note on a scale from 1 to 5 how much you enjoyed eating the food.

3. The Best Exercise for You

It is essential to begin exercise at a level which is not too demanding; otherwise you may find it impossible to keep to a regular plan and are more likely to injure yourself. So it is important first of all to consider whether you are in good basic health, how fit you are, and whether you have a special problem which suggests swimming rather than walking, jogging or the Home Workout as your basic exercise.

Are you in reasonable health?

Sudden unaccustomed exercise can be hazardous. Most at risk is the middle-aged man who has played energetic sports in the past but has become inactive and physically unfit. Not realizing how unfit he is, he may suddenly decide to have an energetic workout or a game of squash. This is the wrong way to begin what is intended to be a steady, long-term programme of exercise and carries a risk of damage to muscles, joints and tendons, if nothing else.

There is no need for most people to consult their doctor before beginning our exercise programme because it begins very gently and everyone can find their own level. However, there are some people who obviously should not follow any exercise programme without discussing it with their doctor first. So check the following questions before you start:

- Have you ever had high blood pressure or heart disease?
- Are you recovering from an illness or operation?

If the answer to either of these questions is yes, then you should discuss whether to start the exercise programme with your doctor. There is considerable evidence that exercise can be helpful in lowering certain common types of high blood pressure and in aiding recovery from a heart attack, but this obviously varies with individual circumstances. Exercise in such cases should be taken only with medical advice.

■ Do you have chest trouble such as asthma or bronchitis?
■ Do you have problems with joint pains, severe back pain, or arthritis?

If you answer yes to either of these questions then discuss undertaking an exercise programme with your doctor. Swimming can be a very beneficial exercise for people who suffer from joint and back problems because it takes the weight off the joints and avoids the jarring movement involved in jogging. Exercise can help such people regain flexibility of movement. Swimming is also the best form of exercise for people who suffer from asthma. Our swimming programme should suit many people with these problems, but discuss it with your doctor first.

■ Are you seriously worried that exercise may affect any aspect of your health?
■ Are you seeing your doctor or some other medical adviser regularly for any reason?

There may be other reasons that you know about which suggest caution in taking exercise. If so, discuss them with your doctor or medical adviser. Exercise can often help people with a chronic medical problem. To take just one example, diabetics often notice improved control of their condition when they take more exercise, but if they are taking insulin they may need to adjust the dose. Exercise can also be a great morale booster for people suffering from depression or anxiety; taking drugs for 'nerves' is certainly no reason for not taking exercise.

If the answer to all these questions is no, then you can go on to select the best exercise plan for your fitness level.

If you have a bad cold, feel feverish or debilitated, then you should put off starting the exercise programme for a day or two until you feel better. If, later on, mild illness interrupts your exercise programme, start again at a lower level – going back a week or even two weeks. With luck you will be back to where you were before in less than a week and in the long run you will progress faster this way.

How Much Exercise

In order to bring about weight loss, exercise should be aerobic. That is, it should be vigorous, raising the pulse and increasing the rate of breathing (though not so strenuous that you cannot hold a conversation while you're exercising); it should also be continuous, lasting uninterrupted for at least 20 minutes.

Exercising three times a week is sufficient if the aim is just to get fit. The lungs and heart will increase in capacity and there will probably be a noticeable improvement in general energy level and in resistance to physical or emotional stress. But if the aim is to become thinner as well as fitter you will have to exercise more often, at least four or five times a week. Exercise should become a part of your daily routine and you should never allow more than one day to go by without exercising unless you are ill. Research has proved that you will lose weight three times faster if you exercise four to

YOUR ABC DIARY	Monday Date / /	Tuesday Date / /	Wednesday Date / /
	Activity/exercise	Activity/exercise	Activity/exercise
Body measurements:			
Date / /	Sleep: hrs	Sleep: hrs	Sleep: hrs
	Behaviour/hunger/emotion	Behaviour/hunger/emotion	Behaviour/hunger/emotion
Chest: Waist:			
Hips: Legs:			
Arms: Weight:			
	Consumption of food	Consumption of food	Consumption of food
Walking: hrs mins miles	Breakfast	Breakfast	Breakfast
Walking/Jogging: hrs mins miles	?Snacks	?Snacks	?Snacks
Swimming: hrs mins lengths	Lunch	Lunch	Lunch
Other exercise:	?Snacks	?Snacks	?Snacks
Total activity: hrs	Evening meal	Evening meal	Evening meal
ABC Road Test: mins mph	?Snacks	?Snacks	?Snacks

five times a week rather than twice a week.

Start by walking

A moderate walking speed is three miles an hour; two miles an hour is slow. The most efficient walking speed, as judged by the army in the First World War, is three and a half miles an hour. Four miles an hour (the speed you must reach to pass the ABC Road Test which follows) is fast, and most people find it impossible to walk faster than five miles an hour. Walking at four miles an hour uses about the same amount of energy as running at the same speed; this is why it is safe to proceed to gentle jogging once you have passed the ABC Road Test.

Many people who are older or unfit may find it difficult to walk at much more than two and a half miles an hour to begin with or to walk for a full half hour. Choose a pace which you find comfortable but invigorating. It is a good idea to go with a friend and talk while you walk so that you are not worrying too much about time and distance. Aim to do a half hour

walk every other day in this preliminary week; this should be on top of any walking you would normally do. If half an hour is too much, walk for a shorter period – even if it is only for 10 minutes to begin with.

---

14 MEN

In California, 14 men, aged from 36 to 54, took up running. They built up their runs to an average of 12 miles a week over two years, having previously taken no exercise at all. Over the two year period their percentage of body fat went down from 21.6 to 18. They were not attempting to lose weight – they were trying to get fit, as part of the Stanford University Heart Disease Prevention Programme, run by Professor Peter Wood.

During these two years the men's consumption of food actually went up by 15 per cent, from an average 2,380 calories to an average 2,747 calories. This is the equivalent of an extra hamburger and bun, or three chocolate éclairs, or a slice of apple pie and cream, every day – and yet they still lost weight.

---

4. The ABC Road Test

The test simply involves measuring your walking speed. To do this you must accurately time how long it takes you to walk a measured two miles – perhaps between landmarks identified on an Ordnance Survey Map or on a scaled city street map. Alternatively, measure out a mile using a car milometer. If you can walk two miles in half an hour without any distress and without excessive tiredness afterwards then you are ready to start in Week One with Jogging 1 or Jogging 2, if you want to, or you can continue with walking, or swimming or, from Week Two onwards, with the Home Workout.

Do not worry if the ABC Road Test is too much for you now; if it is, continue with our walking or swimming programme. If you continue walking, rather than swimming, then test yourself once a week, recording the result in your ABC Diary.

Thursday Date / /	Friday Date / /	Saturday Date / /	Sunday Date / /
Activity/exercise	Activity/exercise	Activity/exercise	Activity/exercise
Sleep: hrs	Sleep: hrs	Sleep: hrs	Sleep: hrs
Behaviour/hunger/emotion	Behaviour/hunger/emotion	Behaviour/hunger/emotion	Behaviour/hunger/emotion
Consumption of food	Consumption of food	Consumption of food	Consumption of food
Breakfast	Breakfast	Breakfast	Breakfast
?Snacks	?Snacks	?Snacks	?Snacks
Lunch	Lunch	Lunch	Lunch
?Snacks	?Snacks	?Snacks	?Snacks
Evening meal	Evening meal	Evening meal	Evening meal
?Snacks	?Snacks	?Snacks	?Snacks

WEEK 1

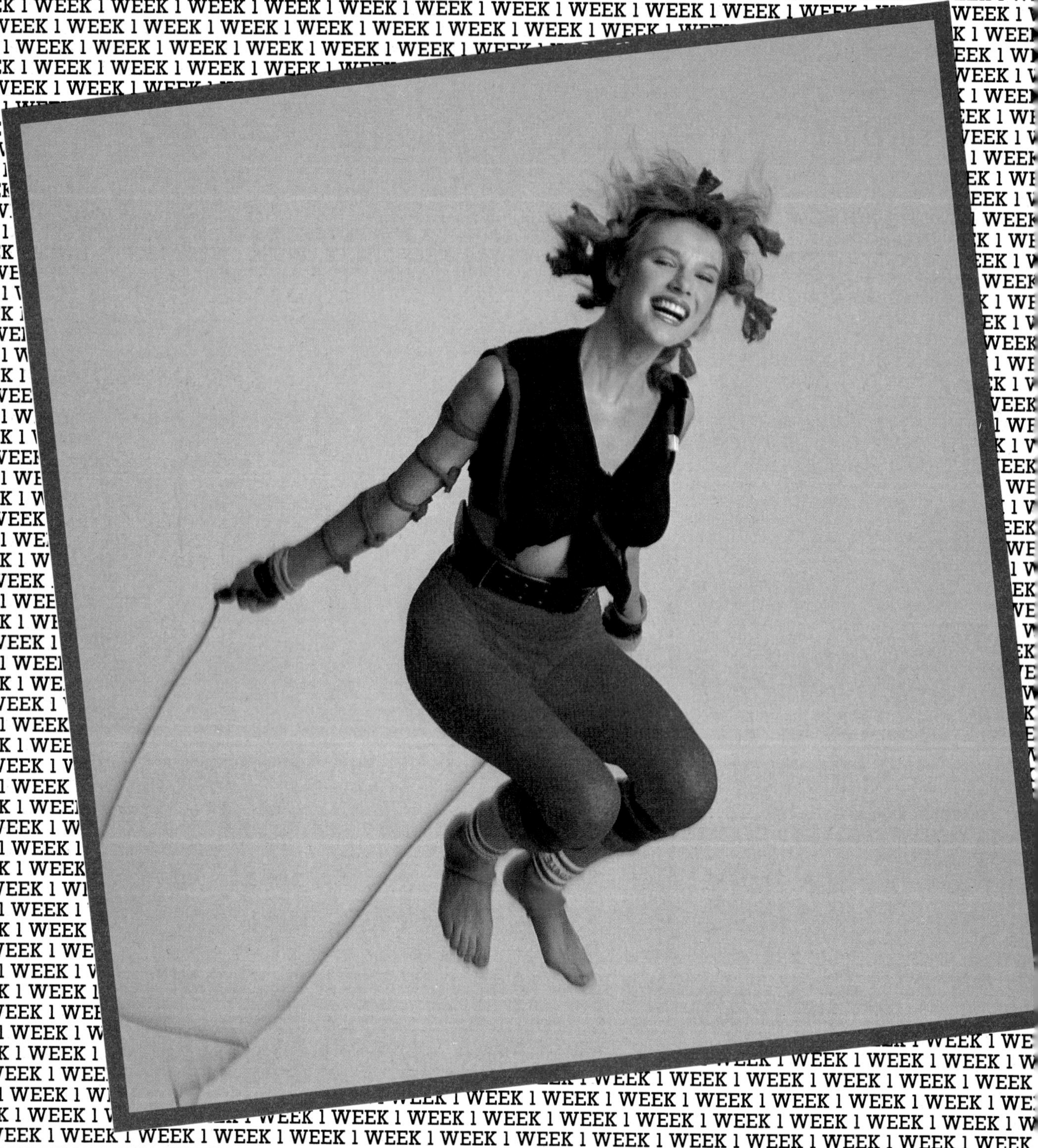

Week 1

A FOR ACTIVITY

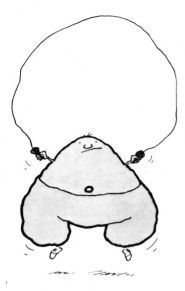

When you have passed the ABC Road Test on page 17 you can begin jogging if you wish; until then continue with the walking programme which follows, or choose one of the two swimming programmes. In Week Two we introduce our Home Workout, but, as this is fairly hard going, we suggest you prepare for it this week with the walking programme.

Some people find it convenient to walk or run before breakfast, and others find exercise a good way of winding down at the end of the day. Whichever time you choose, remember that it is inadvisable to exercise hard for at least an hour after a light meal or two hours after a large meal.

Our programme is carefully graduated for safety, but it is worth knowing some simple warning signs which can be used to assess whether or not you are overdoing it. If you get a pain or tightness in the chest, dizziness, nausea, or loss of muscle control during exercise, stop immediately and consult a doctor. If you find you are still out of breath 10 minutes after taking exercise then you have almost certainly been exercising too hard. The pulse is another guide. Five minutes after exercise it should be down below 120 beats per minute; 10 minutes after exercise it should be below 100.

Do three exercise sessions this week (except Walking Programme – see below)

Walking Programme

Walk briskly for 30 minutes four times this week.
Walking is by far the simplest way of reducing fat. Take the walk at a brisk but comfortable speed. If you find this so tiring that it creates problems for you, then try dividing up the time into three 10-minute walks a day or two 15-minute walks. Remember, though, that this must be in addition to any walking you do normally when going to work or shopping. Old people, or people suffering from an illness which makes walking difficult, may need to start with even shorter walks.

Women who are used to wearing high heels will need to wear flat shoes for comfortable walking. High heels cause an abnormal shortening of the calf muscles, so women who never normally wear anything else may find flat shoes uncomfortable at first. They may also feel some pain in their shins, because the shin muscles are having to work in constant opposition to the powerful and abnormally short calf muscles. Running shoes or similar leisure shoes are ideal for walking. When buying them, make sure that the toes are not cramped.

Your aim should be to raise your walking speed by about half a mile per hour every week or two, or in comfortable stages. In order to judge your progress in training, measure the speed at which you walk by doing the ABC Road Test. You should do the Road Test at the end of each week's training and record the result in your ABC Diary.

Once you have reached four miles an hour you are ready to graduate to Jogging 1 or Jogging 2. When you are getting near to the four-mile-an-hour breakthrough point you may feel you want to start running. If you can run comfortably, do. Get the feel of it gradually; don't rush at it and overtire yourself.

Running Style

Before going on to the jogging programme, here is some general advice on running. First and foremost, it should always feel natural and comfortable.

Do not run on your toes unless you really find this comfortable. Most people tire very rapidly if they run on their toes, and it also puts an unnecessary strain on muscles and tendons.

Most people strike the ground with the heel and outside of the foot first, then rotate on to the ball of the foot while moving forward. The foot moves with a rocking motion until you finally get lift-off at the toe.

OVERWEIGHT PEOPLE ARE LESS ACTIVE

One in four women and one in three men in Britain need to lose weight for health reasons, according to a *Sunday Times* MORI Poll. However, it does not seem to be the greedy eating of extra meals and snacks that makes people overweight. The poll showed that people who are overweight do *not* eat any more often than anyone else and that they are *less* likely than others to take sugar in their tea or coffee. In fact, it is slim women who are most likely to eat snacks – particularly during the morning. They are also more likely to eat chocolate and sweets at any time of the day, presumably because they don't feel they have to hold back.

People who are overweight are, according to the MORI Poll, *less* keen than others on the more active sports such as swimming, squash, tennis, badminton, running, aerobics and keep fit classes. People who are overweight choose less vigorous activities – gardening was often the quoted favourite. Women who are overweight are *more* likely than other women to take no exercise. In fact a quarter of the British population takes *no exercise at all*, although another quarter takes some form of exercise everyday.
MORI interviewed a representative quota sample of 1890 adults aged 15+ face to face in 164 constituencies in Great Britain.

Breathe naturally through your mouth. When running you need a lot of oxygen.

Run with a straight back, keep your head up and look forward into the middle distance. Do not look down at the ground except when it is necessary to avoid potholes. Avoid leaning forward – this makes you overbalance, puts an undue strain on muscles, is tiring and may give you back pain.

Swing your legs forward when running, not out to the side.

Choose a comfortable length and speed of stride that you can maintain.

You don't have to pump your arms hard unless you are climbing a steep hill. Your arms provide you with balance, working in the opposite way to your legs; swing them in a natural rhythm as you run.

Your shoulders should be relaxed, not held up, and you do not need to stick your chest out.

As far as possible try to relax while you are running or walking. If you find your arms getting tense, let them hang down and flop at your sides for a little while. If you

find you are clenching your jaw, let your chin drop and waggle it about. If your neck muscles are tight, try shrugging your shoulders.

Jogging Programme

You will need to wear loose-fitting leisure clothes – a track suit is ideal – and gym, tennis or running shoes. It is most important that your shoes are comfortable; they should be slightly larger than you would normally take to allow for the spread of your foot as you run. It is not necessary to buy the most expensive running shoes. For the distances that you will be covering to begin with, an inexpensive pair will be perfectly satisfactory, so long as they are comfortable.

Whichever plan you choose you should always feel that you are exercising within your capability. Ease up and do less if it feels too strenuous.

To begin with you should choose an area of reasonably level ground for jogging – if that is difficult, then make sure your runs are on slight

downward slopes. Avoid running uphill or down steep slopes to begin with; later on this will be a challenge but it is too difficult at first.

An important rule is that you should be able to hold a conversation or sing without difficulty while you are jogging. If you cannot, you are attempting to go too fast.

Jogging 1 provides an easier start for over 35s. But under 35s who are in doubt about their

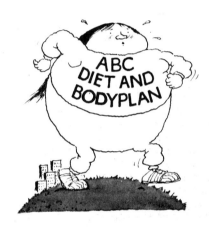

RUNNING SHOES

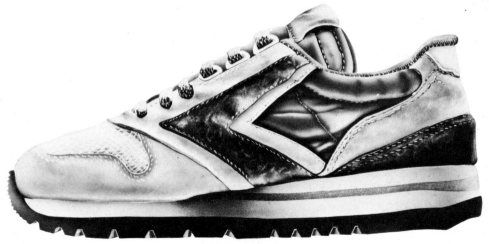

There is a huge variety of running shoes available. These are the points you should look for when buying them:

1. Plenty of material in the sole unit, in more than one layer if possible, to provide good cushioning and flexibility; avoid the ubiquitous

football 'trainer' with a hard, gristly sole.

2. Make sure that the heel is significantly higher than the sole; this is especially important for the beginner runner, whose calf muscles and Achilles tendons need to adjust to a longer 'stretch' than they get from ordinary walking shoes.

3. Remember that the raised heel tab on some models, which serves only to help you pull the shoe on, may irritate the Achilles tendon.

4. Make sure that the shoe is a comfortable fit; don't be influenced by style or a light weight.

ACTIVITY

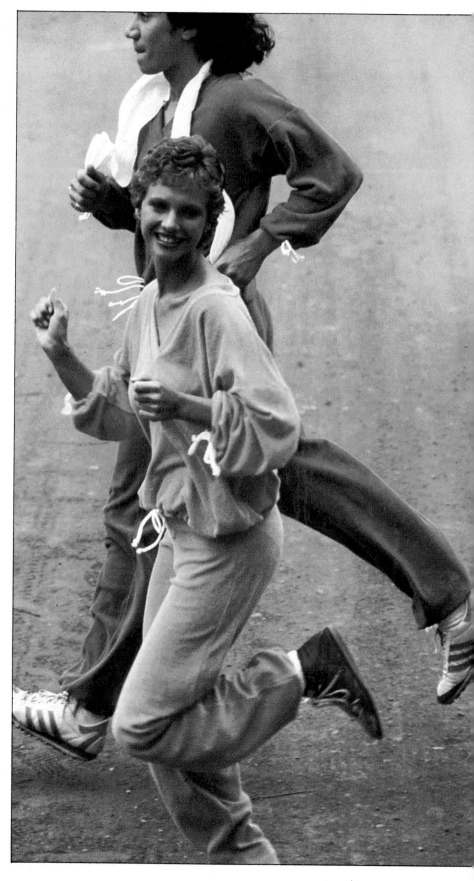

capability and those who take more than two weeks to pass the ABC Road Test should also begin with Jogging 1. This is a mixture of jogging and walking which builds up so that at the end of eight weeks you will be jogging for up to 20 minutes in one session of 30 to 40 minutes.

Most under 35s and fitter over 35s who already take some regular exercise may attempt Jogging 2. Under 35s who do not take any form of exercise which raises a sweat twice a week will probably be happier starting with Jogging 1.

Our jogging programmes start very gently so that you will not injure yourself by putting a strain on unused muscles and tendons. The Cool Down Stretches, which follow Jogging 2, will help prevent muscle soreness and injury. But should you hurt yourself you will find some advice on how to deal with injuries later in the book.

Jogging 1

- Walk briskly for six minutes.
- Jog gently for 30 seconds, then walk briskly for 30 seconds. Do this six times.
- Walk briskly for six minutes.
- Jog gently for 30 seconds, then walk briskly for 30 seconds. Do this six times.
- Walk for six minutes to cool down.
  Total exercise time: 30 minutes.
- Finish with the Cool Down Stretches (which follow Jogging 2).

If the 30 second bursts of jogging are too much for you, find a span of time which is within your capability and work up to 30 seconds.

Jogging 2

- Walk briskly for five minutes.
- Jog for one minute, then walk briskly for one minute. Do this 10 times.
- Walk for five minutes to cool down.
  Total exercise time: 30 minutes.
- Finish with the Cool Down Stretches.

If you find the one minute jogs too much for you, revert to Jogging 1.

Cool Down Stretches

Spend five minutes on these.

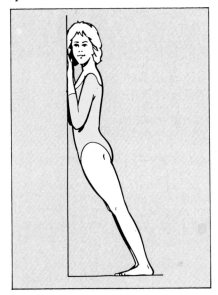

1. Calf Stretch: To help prevent problems with your Achilles tendons you must keep your calf muscles stretched. Stand about two feet away from a wall, and with your body straight gently lean forwards, pressing your palms against the wall and keeping your heels down until you feel the calf muscles stretch. Hold for 30 seconds.

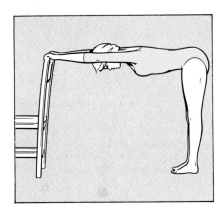

2. Flat Back Stretch: Rest your hands on the back of a chair or table top and walk backwards until your back is parallel to the floor and your legs at right angles to it. This will stretch out your arms and upper back, lower back and hamstrings. Breathe in deeply and exhale slowly as you release. Keep your tummy in.

3. Hamstring Stretch: Depending on how much stretch you felt up the backs of your thighs in the last exercise, use a low chair seat or a table top for this exercise. Keeping your right leg straight rest it on the chair seat or table, knee facing up and hips level. Try to keep the leg you are standing on straight at the same time. Hold for 30 seconds then repeat with the left leg. As you loosen up, use a higher footrest.

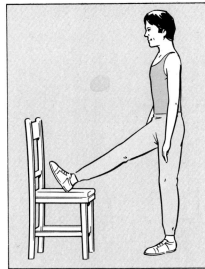

4. Inner Thigh Stretch: Stand with your feet about a yard apart, right foot turned out at right angles to left foot, tummy in and bottom tucked under. Bending your right knee, lunge sideways to the right, feeling the stretch on the left inner thigh. Hold for 30 seconds. Return to centre and repeat with the other leg.

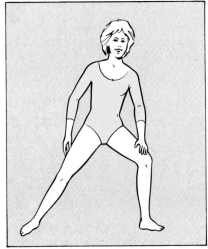

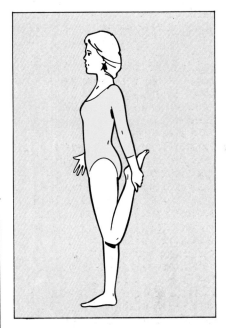

5. Quadriceps Stretch: Rest your left hand on a chair or table top to help with your balance at first. Bend back your right leg and catch hold of the ankle with your right hand. Pull in your tummy and tuck your bottom under. Now gently pull your right knee back until it is in line with your left knee, without arching your back. You will feel the stretch up the front of your thigh (quadriceps). Hold for 30 seconds and repeat with the other leg. You should eventually be able to balance on one leg without holding on to anything.

6. Deep Breathing Stretch: Stand with feet slightly apart, tummy in and bottom tucked under. Breathe in, stretching your arms above your head to a slow count of four. Feel your chest expand. Breathe out, bringing your arms down to your sides, to a slow count of four. Repeat three times.

ACTIVITY

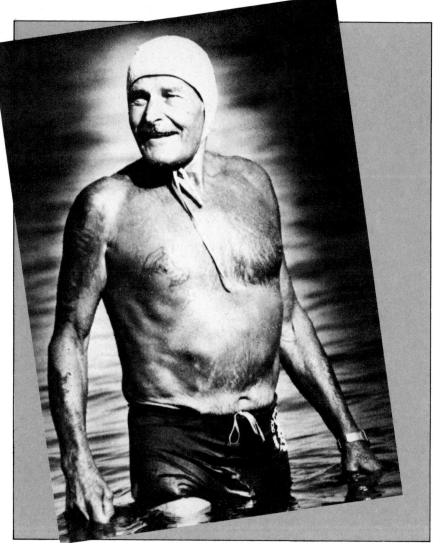

Swimming Programme

Swimming is a first-rate means of getting fit and slim. For people who are overweight or who have stiff joints, it has the great advantage that the water provides support. It is also easier than jogging on the heart, which does not have to pump against gravity during swimming.

Swimming breaststroke or backstroke consumes about the same number of calories as fast walking or slow jogging at four to five miles per hour. Swimming crawl requires more energy and is comparable to a moderately fast squash game or cross-country running. The intensity of your swimming effort also influences the number of calories you burn. A fast breaststroke might use more calories than a slow crawl.

For swimming to be useful as a means of weight reduction, you must be able to do it for half an hour at a time. At first, half an hour will be too long for most people. But you should be able to achieve this length of swim within a few weeks. In the meantime our Pool Exercises, which require no special skills, can be used to increase the amount of work you do and the number of calories you burn.

Technique is obviously important in swimming but for you it will be a secondary consideration. For example, swimmers who have not yet learnt to put their face in the water can still proceed with our programme. We suggest that you try using non-competitive strokes – sidestroke and basic backstroke (backstroke with a sculling movement of the hands underwater, accompanied by 'frog-kicks', as in breaststroke). With these strokes breathing does not have to be synchronised with swimming movements and effort can be concentrated on the stroke itself, enabling you to burn up more energy.

It is important to bear in mind that your swims will probably last less than half an hour to begin with, because you are building up muscles which you have not been using regularly. So make the total exercise time up to half an hour with Pool Exercises or a 15-minute walk straight after your swim if you can, or do some of the home exercises when you get home. Keep a record of the exercise you take in your ABC Diary.

Goggles can be a great help in preventing sore eyes. Get a pair with cellular plastic padding so that they fit snugly around the eyes. A good time to swim, if your pool is open this early, is between 7.00 and 9.00 am, when pools are used only by dedicated swimmers. This is an especially good time to swim if you have been hesitating because of embarrassment at being seen in a swimming costume.

We have devised two swimming plans:

Swimming 1 is for people who are not strong swimmers but can manage at least four lengths of a 25-metre pool and for over-35s who do not take regular exercise or are in doubt about their capability. It includes a set of exercises which require no swimming skill.

People who cannot yet manage four lengths will not be able to build up their exercise to a level which will result in weight loss in the eight-week period of the ABC Bodyplan, so they are advised to follow one of the other exercise plans. However, there may be some people who suffer from joint problems, or who can't take other forms of exercise for some reason and are not strong swimmers.

They can certainly benefit from these programmes but it will take them longer. Their best plan is probably to join a swimming class, or to build up their skills gradually, swimming widths in the shallow end until they can manage four lengths and start this programme. They should also make extra use of our Pool Exercises.

Swimming 2 is for experienced swimmers who can manage two strokes well and are accustomed to regular exercise. If you can swim two lengths without stopping or changing to another stroke, that counts as doing a stroke well. The two strokes might be breaststroke and backstroke, or front crawl and back crawl, but any combination will do.

Swimming 1

Warm-up
■ Swim a few leisurely widths. Use the strokes you know to get used to them again. If possible, include two widths of sidestroke and two widths of basic backstroke.

Exercise
■ Begin with the Pool Exercises (see illustrations).
■ Swim four lengths (25 metres each), alternating your best stroke with sidestroke or basic backstroke.
■ Rest for at least one minute.
■ Repeat sequence of four lengths.
■ End with the Pool Exercises. Rest between lengths to recover your breath if you need to.

Swimming 2

Warm-up
■ Begin with the Pool Exercises (see illustrations).
■ Do two lengths of sidestroke.
■ Do two lengths of basic backstroke.
   Without hurrying, find the best way of getting a strong pull on the water.

Exercise
■ Do six lengths, using your preferred strokes and one other stroke. Use the sidestroke and backstroke lengths to work really hard without worrying about breathing.
■ End with five minutes or more of relaxed swimming.

POOL EXERCISES

These are particularly useful for the slow or hesitant swimmer, because they help to burn up more energy by increasing the amount of aerobic exercise in an enjoyable way. Strong swimmers may prefer just to swim, but these exercises are fun and a challenging way of varying your routine. Beginners may find these exercises quite strenuous; warm up by swimming a few widths before you tackle them.

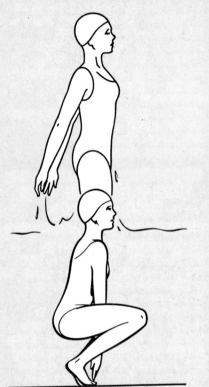

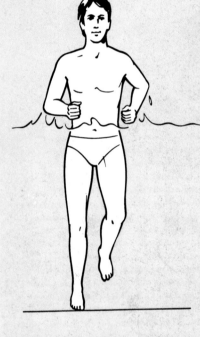

1. Waterjumps: Stand at the shallow end with the water up to your waist, or higher if you like. Bend your knees, touch your feet (perhaps with your head under the water) then jump out of the water as high as possible. Repeat this exercise five to 10 times. Work up to 25 times over the next few weeks.

2. Waterjogs: Run on the spot in the water, bringing your knees as high as possible. Take up to 15 steps with each leg. Work up to 80 steps over the next few weeks.

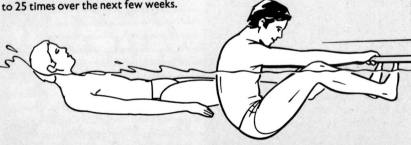

3. Push-offs: Hold on to the edge of the pool and bring the soles of your feet up flat against the side of the pool, between your hands. Then let your hands go and push off with all your strength from the side of the pool.

Make a note of how far you get. Go back to the edge and see if you can do better. Repeat five to 10 times, and work up to 25 times over the next few weeks.

B FOR BEHAVIOUR

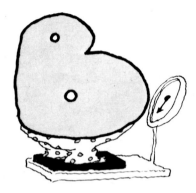

Customs of a lifetime cannot be altered overnight, but psychologists have shown that it only takes three weeks to establish a new habit. By studying your ABC Diary, you can discover what habits you need to change. It should be filled by now with information about what you ate and when, the emotions and events that triggered overeating, and your particular weaknesses. Your answers to the Body Quiz at the beginning of the book will have approximately identified your eating style. You can now use this information to spot habits which are easy to tackle and set about changing them.

Your ABC Diary

A quick glance at your entries may be enough to tell you your main problem (too many unscheduled snacks, for example), and to suggest what your goals should be (to cut down on snacks). Examine your Diary to see which of the following presents the biggest obstacle: irregular eating; not knowing when to stop; eating in response to certain triggers; lack of information. You may find unexpected patterns, or they may fall into easily identifiable categories which suggest immediate goals.

How to Change Your Eating Habits

Ad hoc eating: Do you live on snacks all day, then kid yourself that you've hardly eaten a thing? It is important to eat three meals a day, however small and unconventional. Eat muesli for dinner if you wish. You can have snacks too, but do plan them. If you sample food while you're cooking, limit yourself to a specific amount – say two or three teaspoonsfuls per dish. Leftovers should go straight into a soup, the freezer, the fridge or the bin.

When to stop: Do you eat sensibly and at set times, but then can't stop? Aim to eat more slowly, and avoid second helpings. If particular foods are a problem because you can't eat them in small quantities, keep them out of the house, or at least out of sight for now. In time you should be able to desensitize yourself to them.

Put your finger on the trigger: Find what prompts you to eat then learn to break the link with food. It may be a *feeling.* The ones to track down are those that turn you to food – anxiety, hurt, depression, anger, boredom or excitement. Ban eating for at least an hour after the next bout of anxiety, hurt or whatever. Fight boredom with activity. Relieve stress and anxiety with exercise or relaxation (we'll give more details later). If you are

THE FOOD OF LOVE

Slim women are more likely to feel attractive and less likely to suffer from stress than other women, according to a *Sunday Times* MORI Poll. Slim men, on the other hand, are not likely to feel more attractive and are no less likely to suffer from stress than fatter men. This may be why women are so much keener to lose weight than men, and perhaps why one in five women eats less when they fall in love, while the male appetite remains unaffected by romance.

Nine out of 10 men and women who, according to the MORI Poll, wanted to lose weight thought that excess weight did not hinder romantic life or work. However, one in five of the women thought that excess weight hindered social life, which suggests that being overweight perhaps carries a social stigma. Nevertheless, people who are overweight still have their say. They are, on the whole, less afraid than slimmer friends of expressing their views on matters about which they feel strongly. They are also more inclined than others to be patient and friendly.

Underweight men and women are, it was found, more likely to be moody and tense. About 25 per cent of slim women (and even more skinny women) want to lose weight when they have no need. These women (10 per cent of all women) are, if not actually anorexic, then potentially so. On the other hand very few slim or skinny men are interested in losing weight.

anxious, find out why you feel threatened. Learn to express your anger – but only after you've simmered down enough to be rational and assertive – and calmly to tell your loved ones when they hurt you.

If it is *people* who incite you to over-indulge and they can't be avoided, try to see them at fixed times when you feel strong. Certain *events* may sabotage your good intentions. In restaurants learn to order salad dishes and skip courses, though if you do succumb to the chocolate mousse don't give up altogether. At parties fend off friends who press rich

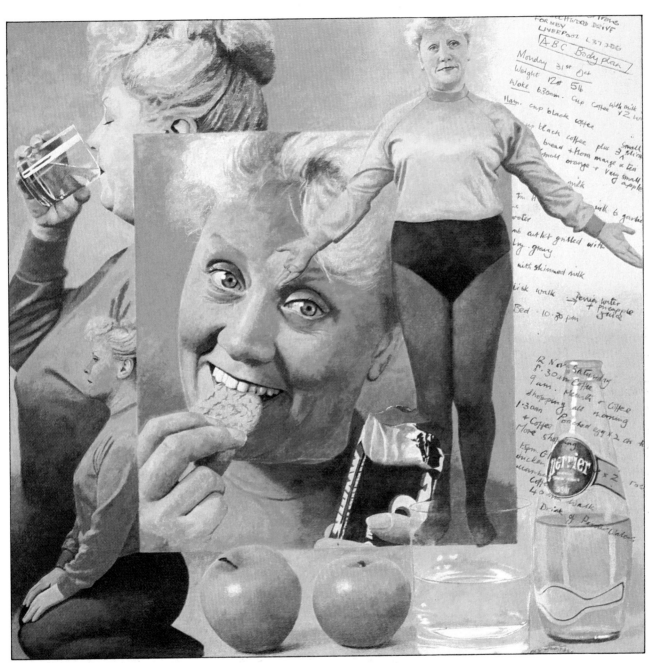

foods and second helpings. Organize a wholesome snack for teatime. Allow yourself treats and try not to distinguish between 'Dieting Me' and 'Non-dieting Me'.

Know your facts: Unless you know which foods are fat-packed or over-sugared and high in calories, you may choose the wrong ones. Many people think cheese and sausages are protein and therefore 'good', without realising that the protein comes with a great deal of fat. Aim to improve your knowledge of food values.

How to change a bad habit

Pinpoint the problem. Look for the weak spots but don't make value judgements. 'I eat 14 snacks a day, when I should eat no more than four apart from meals' is a problem you can start to tackle. 'I gorge myself all day and can't stop' is too vague and depressng.

Set a goal: Make it small, realistic and measurable. 'To drink no more than one glass of wine at lunch today and tomorrow' is better than 'to drink less alcohol'. Start with the easiest goal first, and record

your progress in your ABC Diary. Writing down a target should help to improve your resolve.

Reward yourself: Decide on a gift now and award it to yourself as soon as possible after your goal is achieved. Some people find it particularly hard to reward themselves. Being rewarded ceremoniously is more important then the reward itself, which can be as humble as a magazine you wouldn't normally buy. Self-esteem will increase with every target met.

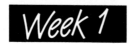

Week 1

C FOR CONSUMPTION

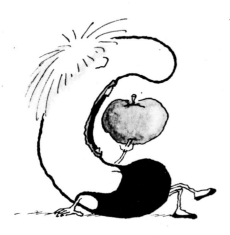

The Constant Energy Diet provides a series of guidelines which you can use to influence your choice of food, whether you cook it for yourself or not. The aim in this first week is to increase the amount of fibre in your diet in order to give you more satisfying bulk; to decrease sugar, which is high in calories and creates rather than assuages appetite; to decrease fat calories because most of us in the West eat too many; and to control alcohol consumption. Begin with our 10 Rules for a Better Diet (see illustration). If you have difficulty following them, do not despair, because each week we will be expanding on some aspect of the Diet, giving detailed information and help. This week we begin with advice for sugar addicts and for people who want to control their alcohol consumption. And for everyone we give advice on how to begin the day with breakfast.

Breakfast

For most of us, our longest stretch without food runs from bedtime to breakfast, and to keep body and mind working effectively, we need to refuel in the morning, when the sugar level in the blood is at its lowest.

Yet one British person in six eats no breakfast, and of the five who do, a quarter eat only toast. Research shows that these people may be working below capacity at the beginning of that day, and that people who eat breakfast perform better than those who skip it. Without breakfast, output, endurance and strength are reduced, reactions slow down and concentration and learning ability are impaired. A study of foundry workers showed that skipping breakfast increased a man's chances of having an accident during the morning.

Warnings to eat breakfast often fall on deaf ears however. 'If I eat breakfast, I'm ravenous by 11 o'clock' ... 'Just the thought of

---

SLIMMING AND YOU

The most popular and effective way of slimming is not to count calories – the method most often recommended by experts. Most slimmers find it easier simply to cut back on their food intake or to cut certain foods out of the diet completely. These were the methods preferred by more than half of a representative sample of 600 slimmers who were interviewed in *The Sunday Times* MORI Poll on weight and exercise. The ABC Diet and Bodyplan makes use of this popular and effective cutting-back method.

Only one in 10 men and women attempt to slim by counting calories – whereas one in two slimmers are prepared to cut back on their food intake in general. Eating smaller portions at meal times is used by one in three slimmers and is one of the most effective ways of slimming, according to those who tried it. Cutting down on snacks is also a popular and effective method. Cutting out courses and missing meals – which we do not recommend – were generally the least popular and least effective ways of slimming according to the poll.

One out of two slimmers also finds that cutting out sweet or fatty foods is an effective way of slimming. One in seven male slimmers finds that cutting down on alcoholic drinks is effective in reducing weight, but fewer women find this effective, perhaps because they are less likely to be drinking regularly in the first place. Cutting down on starchy foods – which we do not recommend – was also found to be an effective way of slimming. However it is healthier and more efficient to slim by cutting down on sugars and fats, as we suggest in the Constant Energy Diet.

Exercise was used as a way of losing weight by one in three of the female slimmers polled but, surprisingly, by only one in six male slimmers. As many men took exercise but they did not acknowledge that they did it in order to lose weight. Over half of those who used exercise for slimming found it effective – so giving strong popular support for the concept behind the ABC Bodyplan. Jogging, weight-training and keep-fit were judged to be the most effective forms of exercise for slimmers by those who tried them.

EFFECTIVENESS OF VARIOUS METHODS OF SLIMMING

Method	% of slimmers who tried method	% of slimmers who found it effective
Eating a limited number of calories a day	15	56
Cutting back on food in general	45	62
Taking smaller portions at meal times	30	58
Cutting out some snacks	21	52
Cutting out courses from meals	9	47
Missing meals	8	37
Avoiding certain foods/drinks	49	68
Taking more exercise	30	57

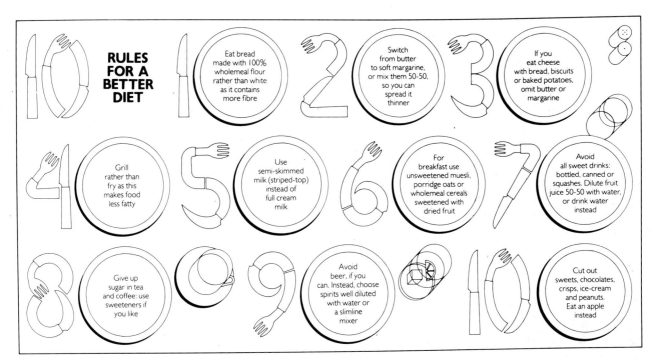

RULES FOR A BETTER DIET

1 Eat bread made with 100% wholemeal flour rather than white as it contains more fibre

2 Switch from butter to soft margarine, or mix them 50-50, so you can spread it thinner

3 If you eat cheese with bread, biscuits or baked potatoes, omit butter or margarine

4 Grill rather than fry as this makes food less fatty

5 Use semi-skimmed milk (striped-top) instead of full cream milk

6 For breakfast use unsweetened muesli, porridge oats or wholemeal cereals sweetened with dried fruit

7 Avoid all sweet drinks: bottled, canned or squashes. Dilute fruit juice 50-50 with water, or drink water instead

8 Give up sugar in tea and coffee: use sweeteners if you like

9 Avoid beer, if you can. Instead, choose spirits well diluted with water or a slimline mixer

10 Cut out sweets, chocolates, crisps, ice-cream and peanuts. Eat an apple instead

breakfast makes me feel ill' ... 'It's bad enough having to get to work, without thinking about breakfast; besides, I'm just not hungry' are common ripostes.

A few people do seem to get by without eating in the morning, but this is not recommended for anyone who has trouble controlling their eating. Regular meals train the body to expect food at set times and greatly weaken the urge to binge, which strikes after long periods without food. Hence the WeightWatchers slogan 'Never never skip a meal'.

The overweight often bypass breakfast, leave out lunch or eat lightly at midday and concentrate their eating on the evening meal. The drawbacks to this are both physiological and psychological. It is bad for their heart, their willpower and their weight. Far better to follow the old adage: 'Breakfast like a king, lunch like a prince and dine like a pauper'.

If less than three meals a day are eaten, cholesterol levels in the blood show a tendency to rise. So do levels of the dangerous fats known as triglycerides. In the long term this increases the risk of heart disease. At the same time glucose (sugar) tolerance is lowered, so that the body is less able to keep the level of sugar in the blood stable. When this sugar

level drops, hunger and weakness follow.

Research has shown that the person who eats three meals a day is less likely to put on fat than the person who eats the same number of calories at a single sitting, especially in the evening.

By missing breakfast, you're avoiding food at a time when self-control is high (in the morning and early afternoon) and eating more when resistance is lowest (in

the evening). When the time for dinner comes, the body is famished and control goes by the board. And overweight people rarely stop at dinner. Their leisure activities are also likely to culminate in eating, and this regular refuelling may continue unabated until bedtime.

Not eating all day leads dieters to think they deserve a reward for their self-denial. And the reward isn't celery sticks.

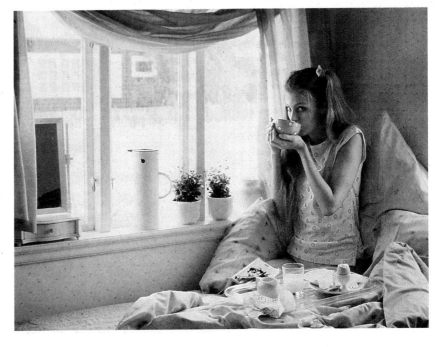

CONSUMPTION

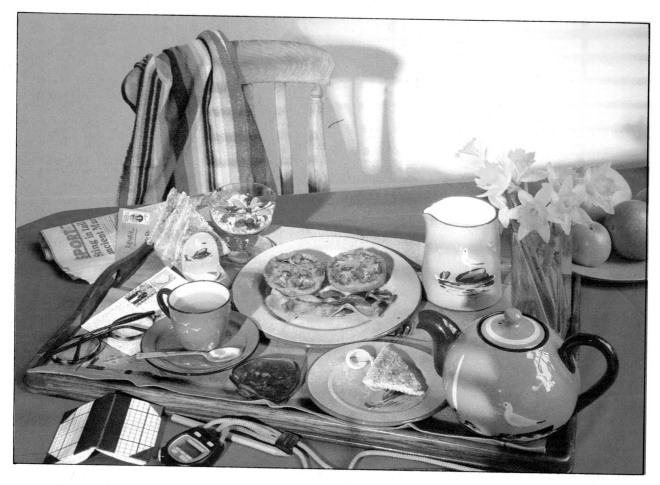

What to eat for breakfast

One of the best breakfast foods is oats, eaten as porridge or muesli. The fibre that oats contain is viscous, which makes it doubly beneficial. Because of it, oats are digested and absorbed more slowly than cereals such as wheat or corn, and therefore help to delay the return of hunger pangs. And this viscous fibre is also particularly good for the heart, sharply reducing cholesterol levels.

When milk is added to any food, glucose sugar enters the blood more slowly, so that adding milk or yoghurt to your oats will keep you satisfied even longer.

To sweeten porridge, add one dessertspoon of sultanas for each person during cooking, or add half a fresh banana or a teaspoon of low-sugar or sugar-free preserve after cooking. Whole Earth make a delicious range of sugar-free preserves (but they must be refrigerated after opening).

Robertsons make a range of jams called Today's Recipe which contain only 50 per cent sugar instead of the usual 67 per cent. You can buy sugar-free muesli at supermarkets or health food stores. Or make this recipe, which can easily be adapted to provide variety.

Muesli

1 lb (450g) rolled oats (preferably 8 oz jumbo oats and 8 oz ordinary oats)
4 oz (100-125 g) chopped walnuts, hazelnuts or almonds
1 oz (25 g) chopped dates
3 oz (75 g) raisins or sultanas
2 oz (50 g) sunflower seeds (or more nuts)
½ oz (12 g) toasted sesame seeds (or more nuts)
¼ tsp zest of orange (use fine grater)
1 tsp cinnamon

Mix ingredients and store in airtight container away from light. Chopped fresh fruit or soaked dried fruit can be added at the table. (Muesli was intended by its originator, Dr Bircher-Benner of Zurich, to be principally a fruit dish). Serve with semi-skimmed milk, low-fat yoghurt, cottage cheese or a mixture of these. For variety, sprinkle over 2 tsp toasted wheatgerm and a pinch of shredded

coconut. For a crunchier texture, spread the mixture on to a baking tray and roast for 15 minutes at Gas Mark 4 (350°F, 180°C).

As an alternative to oats, have a wholemeal cereal – Puffed Wheat, Weetabix, Shreddies, or, best of all, Shredded Wheat, which releases its energy more slowly than the others. Avoid All-Bran because the high phytate content of bran could deplete the body of essential minerals. Bran is best eaten in its integral form, in bread or wholemeal products. Cornflakes are a poor breakfast food because they are digested so quickly that they are not sustaining.

Cooked breakfasts

If you want a cooked breakfast other than porridge, base it on wholemeal bread and avoid fried food. Poached egg, grilled tomatoes or baked beans on toast are possibilities. Baked beans have been criticized because they contain added sugar, but this is offset by the fact that the beans themselves release their energy slowly, as well as being nutritious and high in valuable fibre. Alternatives are grilled bacon, sardines (well drained) or grilled grated cheese on toast, but don't butter the toast because these foods contain enough fat already. The best wholemeal bread is made the old-fashioned way using the full yeast-rising process, rather than the quick aeration process. The full process not only makes a tastier, firmer loaf but destroys more of the potentially harmful phytate.

The Sugar Trap

Many experiments have shown that animals such as rabbits and rats consume more food when they eat sugar. For example, rats given a sugar solution as well as their ordinary food ate 20 per cent more calories. All the evidence points to the conclusion that sugar does not satisfy hunger, as is often thought, but creates it.

People become hungry when their blood sugar falls or when the uptake of sugar from the blood into tissues is blocked by a drug. Sugar in the blood commonly falls below normal levels about an hour after sweet foods have been eaten, creating new hunger. This is because sugar in food stimulates the secretion of insulin, which then rapidly removes sugar from the blood.

Paula Geiselman and Donald Novin, psychologists at the University of California, have looked into the mass of evidence concerning sugar consumption, hunger and obesity. They conclude that a vicious cycle of carbohydrate craving follows the eating of sugar and that this leads to excess intake and weight gain. The Constant Energy Diet is specially formulated to avoid this trap.

The average British person eats around 400 calories' worth of sugar a day – about one-seventh of their daily calorie consumption. But some eat much more: sugar may amount to over a quarter of their daily calorie consumption. Sugar has no nutritive value – it does not provide any vitamins or minerals and can be cut out of the diet completely without any penalty. Cutting down is of positive benefit, because sugar causes bad teeth and diabetes and possibly contributes to the risk of heart disease.

Understanding where the sugar in our diet comes from is an important part of our slimming plan. It is valuable to increase your knowledge of the quantities of sugar which are added to prepared foods, so that you can reduce your intake of nutritionally empty calories.

Everyone knows that jam is largely sugar (69 per cent), but less obvious sources include: drinking chocolate (74 per cent), Ribena (61 per cent), ketchup (23 per cent), biscuits (25-30 per cent) and cakes (up to 50 per cent). Some breakfast cereals are more than half sugar, which makes them sweeter than certain types of chocolate.

A heaped teaspoon of sugar contains about 30 calories, so a person who drinks six cups of tea or coffee a day, each with one teaspoon of sugar, is consuming 180 calories. Soft drinks such as Seven-Up, Tango or Coca Cola contain the equivalent of at least four teaspoons of sugar each.

Our taste for sugar has developed during the course of human evolution, probably as a way of telling us when fruit is ripe and best to eat. But it is only during the last hundred years that sugar has been extracted from cane and beet on a massive scale – and has become a common cause of health problems, including obesity. Sugar, in the purified form with which we are familiar, is unknown in nature. Even brown sugar is a highly purified product, and although some prefer it because of its taste it is just as likely to cause health problems if taken in excess.

A ripe apple contains only about 12 per cent of sugar, an orange 9 per cent and a banana 16 per cent – much less in percentage terms than a biscuit, cake or many other prepared foods. The sugar in fruit is encased in the fibrous structure of the flesh and is released slowly; furthermore, sugar in fruit is mostly of a type called fructose, which is converted more slowly by the body into energy. Therefore fruit is a good way of satisfying a

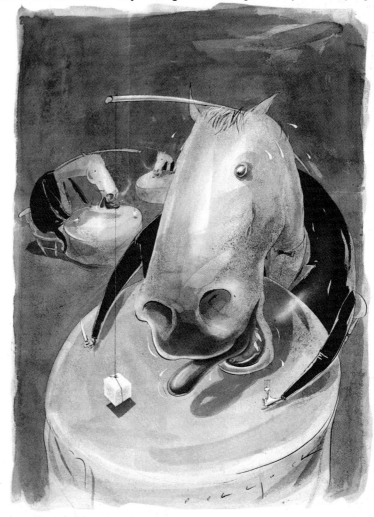

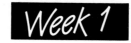

CONSUMPTION

taste for sweet things. If you cut out six teaspoons of sugar a day you can eat two medium apples and a banana without consuming extra calories – and of course the fruit will be much more filling and nutritious.

The 'quick energy' myth

Sugar and sweet manufacturers promote sugar as a source of quick energy, but eating sugar is also a quick way of increasing body fat. A diabetic in insulin shock or a runner at the end of a marathon may get some short-term benefit from a rapid intake of sugar. But in most people sugar triggers a surge of insulin, which rapidly removes sugar from the blood to store it as fat, and within an hour there is generally less sugar in the blood than before the extra sugar was taken. This may well lead to tiredness and a hunger for more sweet food.

Eating sugar before an athletic event probably confers little benefit; indeed, because of the disturbance to the level of insulin in the blood it may even be counterproductive. The body contains its own supply of rapid energy-producing material in the liver in the form of glycogen, a type of starch. There is in fact enough energy stored in the liver for a trained athelete to run a marathon.

How to reduce your sugar intake

Some people who have great determination find they are able to give up something easily once they have decided to do so. If you come into that category all you have to do is to give up sugar in all drinks, and choose carbonated mineral waters such as Perrier or Highland Spring, or tap water, instead of soft drinks and squashes. For those who do find it more difficult, we recommend the following course of action.

Begin by replacing sugar in drinks with saccharin, aspartame˙ (Canderel or NutraSweet) or acesulfame potassium (Hermesetas Gold). Drink low-calorie soft drinks or squashes. This means that you will get an immediate reduction in calorie intake without having to change your taste for sweet things. At the same time set yourself a target of two or three

weeks in which to give up sweeteners altogether, and week by week reduce the amount you take in drinks.

Stop buying biscuits, sweets and chocolates, and stock up on fruit and vegetables instead. Eat fresh fruit instead of gâteau or cheesecake. Bake teabreads and fruit loaves, which generally contain much less sugar than cakes. If you must have cakes, make your own, using half the quantity of sugar given in standard recipes.

Read the labels on all the foods you buy. Ingredients are generally listed in order of quantity. If sugar is the first, second or third ingredient, the product is a very sweet one and should be avoided. Jam, ketchup, chutneys or pickles, though sweet, are used in relatively small quantities combined with other foods, so their sugar content should not necessarily stop you from using them; just be careful about the quantity. Watch out for manufacturers who use various different kinds of sweeteners, such as honey and corn syrup, as well as sugar. If sugar is the fourth ingredient, and honey and corn syrup come next, when counted together these ingredients might make sugar ingredient number one or two.

How to Lose Weight and Carry on Drinking

The Constant Energy Diet does not depend in any way on counting the calories in food. But alcohol is different. Drinking involves social and personal pressures that are quite separate from the appetite for food, and paying special attention to the calorie content of drinks is one good strategy to ensure that your drinking does not jeopardise the gains you make from efforts in other areas. We suggest several other strategies below, but first you should consider whether your drinking is a problem in itself which may require more than calorie counting to sort out. Answer the questions in The Drinking Test honestly, to see if you are drinking too much.

If you are a frequent social drinker, here are a number of ploys you can use to reduce your calorie intake from alcohol.

1. Cut down on the *number of times* a week you go to a bar. Meet friends at a restaurant or café, or at the swimming pool or sports field instead.
2. Always order the *smallest possible measure* – never doubles or pints. If all your friends are drinking pints, develop a taste for bottled beer so that you can drink smaller quantities.
3. *Miss out a round* when you can. Even if you drink vodka, which contains little else besides alcohol and water, you are still downing calories because alcohol itself contains seven calories per gram.
4. If you find it difficult to refuse, ask for a *non-alcoholic drink,* for example a Virgin Mary (straight tomato cocktail), tonic water (preferably slimline) with a slice of lemon, or just soda water with a squeeze of lemon.
5. Always *dilute spirits* with a mixer so that the drink lasts longer, and use all the mixer. A long drink takes longer to drink. When serving wine at a meal, serve water as well, since wine creates thirst and if water is not available you may drink more wine than you want.
6. *Avoid salty foods* such as peanuts or crisps while drinking. They are high in calories and the salt will make you thirsty. If you are hungry, have a sandwich.
7. Go for drinks that are *low in calories.* In general this means the drier and/or less alcoholic drinks (see A Brief Guide to the Calorie Content of Drinks).

A Brief Guide to the Calorie Content of Drinks

Spirits: The spirit with the lowest number of calories is vodka; in fact it is one of the lowest calorie alcoholic drinks of all considered on a calories-per-drink basis – 50 cals per pub measure (1/6 gill). Gin, brandy, rum and whisky contain five calories per measure more. However it is not a good habit to drink spirits unless they are well diluted with a mixer – choose a slimline mixer if you want to keep the calories down.

Aperitifs: Dry sherries such as Harveys Manzanilla or Croft's Delicado or Lysander dry come in at 50 cals per measure (1/3 gill). The dry aperitifs such as Campari (standard measure 1/6 of a gill), Cinzano extra dry (1/3 gill), Riccadonna extra dry Vermouth (1/3 gill), Scotsmac medium dry (1/3 gill) come in at about 55 calories.

Beers: It is better to avoid beers because, apart from the alcohol they contain, they have a lot of maltose sugar, which raises the blood sugar (glucose) faster than any other sugar. Drinking beer overloads the body with sugar, causing a lot of insulin to be secreted into the blood. This is followed within an hour or two by an overshoot – too much sugar is removed from the blood and hunger follows rapidly.
The lowest calorie beer – which is definitely not for serious drinkers – is Barbican alcohol-free lager at 50 cals per 275 ml bottle. Other beers providing 75 cals or less per 275 ml bottle or half pint are: Heldenbrau, Hemeling, Newcastle Amber Ale, Toby Brown Ale, Toby Light Ale, Truman "S", Whitbread Light Ale, Whitbread Party King, Younger's sweet stout.

Wines: Most wines deliver 75 cals or more per 113 ml glass – the same as the lowest calorie beers. However the sweet wines generally deliver a lot more – up to 100 cals per glass. Lowest in calories, at 60-65 per glass, are Real Sangria white and Rosentor's Leitwein. Mosel Spezial and Pedrotti Bianco are also low at around 70 cals per glass. In general the dry German white wines such as the Rieslings and Moselles – particularly the Saar and Ruhr wines of QbA or Kabinett quality – are low in calories. Try also Vinho Verde or dry Muscadet. If you prefer red go for the wines of the Loire such as Bourgueil, Chinon, and red Saumur.

THE DRINKING TEST

1. Do you drink more in order to get drunk than for other reasons? ... YES/NO

2. Do you regularly slip away for a mid-morning drink? ... YES/NO

3. Are you fairly frequently the worse for drink in mid-week? ... YES/NO

4. Do you get drunk alone? ... YES/NO

5. Do you have memory lapses about what you have said or done while drinking? ... YES/NO

6. Do you find that the other people you are drinking with are rather slow in drinking up their rounds? ... YES/NO

7. Do you usually have at least a couple of drinks to help you face a difficult problem? ... YES/NO

If your answer is YES to two or more of these questions then you are probably drinking too much, and should stop drinking for about six months. You should never start drinking heavily again. If you cannot control your drinking seek advice from Alcoholics Anonymous.

YOUR ABC DIARY: Week One					Starting date:			
	WALKING		JOGGING/ WALKING		SWIMMING		HOME WORKOUT	OTHER EXERCISE (e.g. cycling)
	Mins	Miles*	Mins	Miles*	Mins	Lengths	Mins	Mins
Monday								
Tuesday								
Wednesday								
Thursday								
Friday								
Saturday								
Sunday								
TOTAL								

* approximate distance, optional

ABC ROAD TEST	mins		mph					
BODY MEASUREMENTS	Date / /	Chest	Waist	Hips	Arms	Legs	Weight	

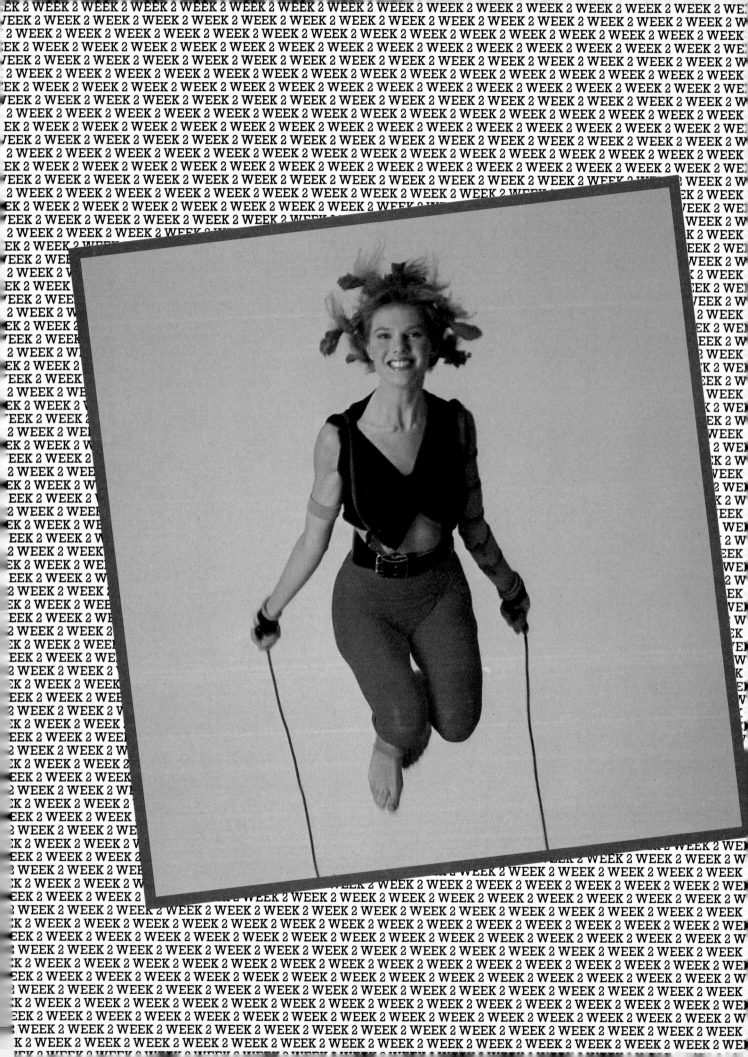

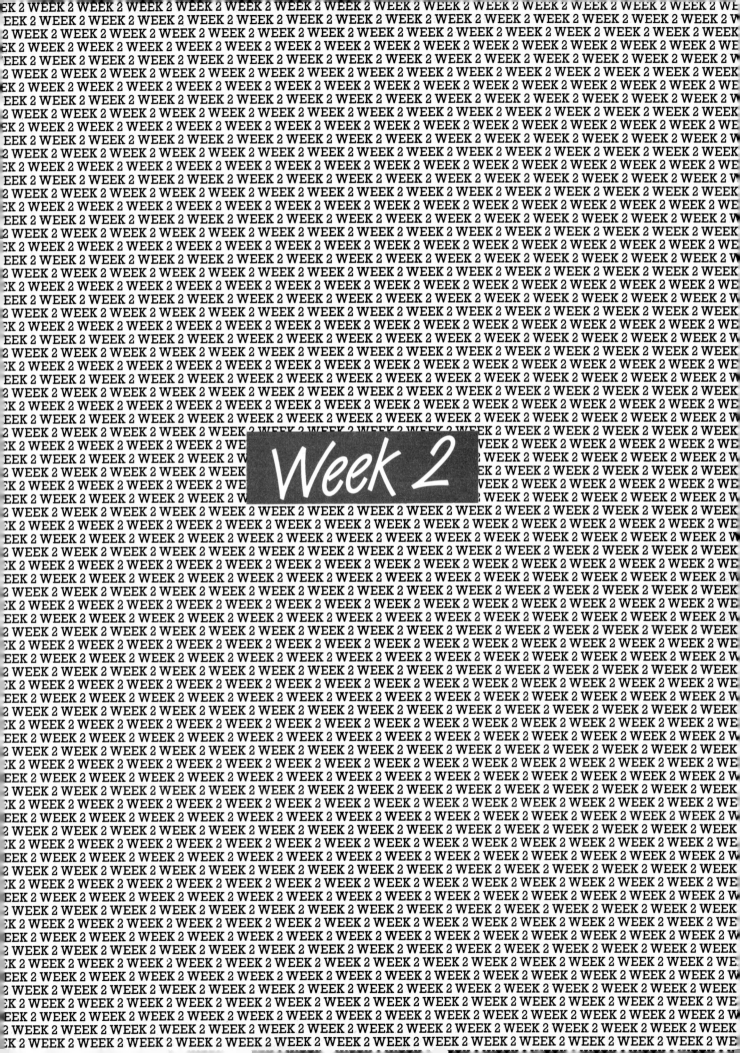

Week 2

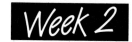

Week 2

A FOR ACTIVITY

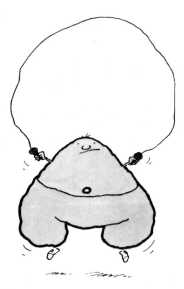

Two weeks is too short a time in which to observe much weight loss; fitness must be increased before really vigorous fat-mobilizing exercise can be taken. If your weight was tending to increase, the first effect of the exercise in Week One may have been to stabilize it. Now your weight should begin to drop.

Our exercise plans are carefully devised to give beginners guidance about how much exercise to take and what to expect from it. However, it is most important to 'listen' to your own body. Soreness of muscles is completely normal and nothing to worry about, but if you find that your exercise is leading to cumulative tiredness you should reduce it. Probably, though, you will find you have more energy.

This week our Home Workout begins. This may be done four or five times a week and could be the only form of exercise taken, or it may be combined with any of the other programmes.

Do four exercise sessions this week (except Walking Programmes – see below).

Walking Programme

Walk briskly for 30 minutes five times this week.
This plan makes increasing demands upon your body as you become fitter. During Week Two try to improve your speed by walking at a brisker pace. Repeat some of the routes you took in Week One, and see if you can cover them more quickly or if you can walk a bit further in the same time. If your muscles feel a bit sore or stiff by now, don't worry: this is a good sign that your body is beginning to respond to the extra work it is doing.

Try to include more walking in your daily routine. Get off the bus a stop or two earlier on your way to work or the shops. If you already walk to work, take a different and longer route. (This may mean leaving a second pair of shoes to wear at work.) When it is difficult for you to get out of the house or the weather is bad, do the Home Workout, which starts this week, instead.

Jogging Programme

Sprains and strains
If you develop a sprain, or painful joints and muscles, stop the daily programme and do not exercise the following day. If the sprain or strain has diminished after 48 hours, begin again with a reduced programme. You may be able to resume gentle jogging, or you may prefer to replace jogging with walking or swimming until you feel ready to go back to the full programme.

Minor injuries involving tendons or muscles heal better if the injured part is kept moving. Even with minor sprains (injuries to ligaments) it is advisable to return to normal activity within a few days. However, if an injury or pain is worse after a day, or has not lessened after 48 hours, you may wish to seek medical advice. Although painful, these injuries are not medical emergencies, and generally no harm will result from delaying a visit to the doctor. You should be guided by the severity of your pain in deciding whether or not to seek medical advice.

Jogging 1
■ Walk briskly for six minutes.
■ Jog gently for one minute then walk for one minute. Do this three times.
■ Walk briskly for six minutes.
■ Jog gently for one minute then walk for one minute. Do this three times.
■ Walk for six minutes to cool down.
Total exercise time: 30 minutes
■ Finish with the Cool Down Stretches (see Week One).

Work within your capability; if you feel out of breath during your one minute jog you should recover during the walk. If you feel exhausted, stay with the Week One programme a little longer.

Jogging 2
■ Walk briskly for two minutes.
■ Jog for two minutes, then walk for one minute. Do this three times.
■ Walk briskly for eight minutes.
■ Jog for two minutes, then walk for one minute. Do this three times.
■ Walk for two minutes to cool down.
Total exercise time: 30 minutes
■ Finish with the Cool Down Stretches (see Week One).

You have now greatly increased your jogging time, but do not be tempted to overdo it, because your body needs time to adapt to these new demands.

Swimming Programme

Swimming 1
Warm-up
■ Do four widths of the pool, alternating side stroke and basic backstroke.
Your aim is to develop a confident sidestroke and basic backstroke. Concentrate on getting into an easy rhythm.
Exercise
■ Begin with the Pool Exercises (see Week One).
■ Aim to swim 10 lengths (25 metres each), changing your stroke after each length (for example, breaststroke followed by sidestroke). Rest between

lengths until your breathing becomes steady.
■ Repeat the Pool Exercises.
■ End with a few minutes of slow swimming or floating to wind down.

Swimming 2
Warm-up
■ Swim two slow lengths (25 metres each) of any stroke. Practise regular breathing and concentrate on getting a good pull through the water.
Exercise
■ Begin with the Pool Exercises (see Week One).
■ Swim 16 lengths, changing strokes with each length. Use sidestroke or basic backstroke in addition to your preferred strokes if you wish, in order to work harder without getting breathing problems.
Total: 18 lengths
■ End with the Pool Exercises.

The Home Workout

The Home Workout is designed for the average reasonably active person who really wants to lose weight. It is flexible enough to be adapted to varying levels of fitness. People over 35 who have sedentary jobs and are not accustomed to exercise may find the full Workout difficult to achieve in the early stages. If you find this, do one cycle (steps 1 to 4) of the Workout, which takes about 15 minutes, and take a 15 minute walk. For maximum effect the walk should come immediately before or after the Workout.

The exercises are ordered so that your body is warmed up steadily, working all the major muscle groups and exercising the heart and lungs.

First, change into loose clothes. You can do all the exercises in bare feet if you want to, except for skipping, which should be done in gym shoes or running shoes to protect your toes. Lively music will help you establish a rhythm.

Do the Home Workout three times during the week plus one or two 40 minute walks.

The Home Workout consists of four parts, which are repeated to

take a total of half an hour, followed by a five-minute cool down.
1. Warm Up Exercises (see illustration) – five minutes.
2. Dancing or room running (see below) – five minutes.
3. Skipping (see below) – two and a half minutes.
4. Stair Climbing (see below) – two and a half minutes.
5. Repeat steps 1 to 4.
Total exercise time: 30 minutes.
6. Do the Cool Down Stretches (see Week One).

Warm Up Exercises

Start by standing with your feet apart, your tummy in, buttocks tightened and tucked under. Don't spend more than five minutes on these exercises.

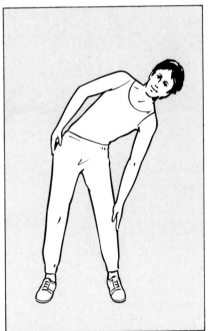

Side Bends. Keeping your buttocks tucked under and tightened, lift and bend the top half of your body over to the right and reach down the side of your leg. Do not allow your hips to push out to the side and do not lean backwards or forwards. Feel the stretch up the left side of your body. Make eight small, smooth reaching movements, then lift and repeat to the left, feeling the stretch this time up the right side. Now repeat the sequence.

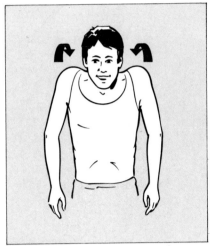

Shoulder Movements. Lift your shoulders towards your ears, then relax them down. Do this four times. Bring the shoulders forwards, lift them up, pull them back and relax them down. Continue moving your shoulders in backward circles, speeding up the repeats.

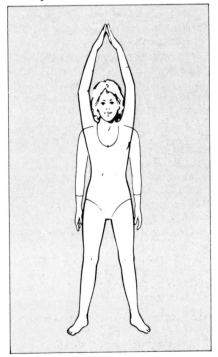

Arm Circles. Swing your right arm round and back in a circle four times, brushing the side of your head with your arm each time. Then do this four times with your left arm, then eight times with both arms together, making sure your back doesn't arch as the arms swing back.

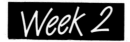

A C T I V I T Y

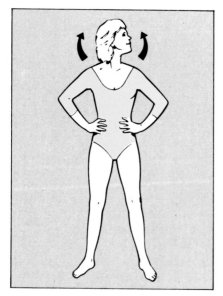

Head Movements. Relax and drop your shoulders and tuck in your chin. Tilt your head forwards slowly, stretching the muscles at the back of your neck. Then bring your head back up, keeping your shoulders down. Do this four times. Tilt your head over to the right; make a slow forward semi-circle to the left and back again. Do this four times.

Twists. In this exercise only the top half of your body turns, so do not allow your hips to turn and do not lean backwards or forwards. Tighten your buttocks. Put your arms out to the side. Look over your right shoulder and, using smooth movements, twist your top half round to the right and back to centre eight times. Repeat to the left. Then repeat the whole sequence.

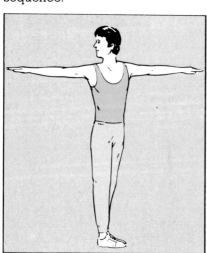

Knees to Chest. Clasp your right knee and pull it towards your chest without bending forwards. This will help to release lower back and hamstring muscles. Hold for a few seconds, then do the same with your left leg. Work each leg eight times. Now, increase the stretch by bringing your forehead towards your knee as you pull it upwards. This will also improve your balance. Work each leg eight times.

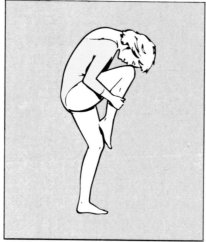

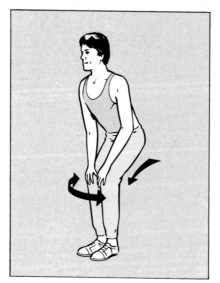

Knee and Calf Releases. Bring your feet together and put your hands on your knees. Bend your knees, keeping your heels on the floor. Providing you have not had any knee injuries, circle both knees together to the right eight times, then to the left eight times (keep them in the bent position), then bounce forwards eight times.

HOW TO IMPROVISE YOUR OWN DANCE ROUTINE

If you are not sure how to begin your own dance routine in the Home Workout, here are some suggestions which should suit both men and women. Play some music with a strong beat at a moderate speed. When you have got used to the following movements continue to do them without any straining to a quicker beat. Remember the aim is to get a good even pace going so that you get aerobic exercise. However, remember that you should be able to talk to a friend or sing while you are doing it.

1. Walk sideways to the left following the rhythm of the music, clapping to the beat as you go. Take four to eight steps and walk back again. Do this six times. This should get you used to the rhythm.

2. Now stand with your feet together. Make one step sideways to the right and then bring your left foot over to it. At the same time move your right arm in a circular movement out front, around and back to your side. Then move your left foot back and bring the right foot to join it, making the same circular movement with the left hand. Now move from left to right in rhythm to the music.

3. Place your feet wide apart and bend your knees. Push your bottom out behind and your arms out in front. Then do the opposite: bring your hips forward and your shoulders back. Do this 16 times to the music.

4. Stand with your feet together. Swing your arms up to the sides and at the same time bend your knees. Straighten your knees, let your arms swing back down, then repeat the movement.

5. Now jump for joy! First to the left, clapping your hands while you are in the air. Smile as you are doing it. Then jump to the right, clap and smile. Repeat several times.

6. Put your arms straight above your head. Sway them to the left and, at the same time, lift your right foot off the ground, straighten, and sway to the other side, lifting your left foot off the ground. Get a good rhythm going to the music.

7. Try some dance push-ups to the music – but not the kind you do on the floor. Stand with your legs apart, push up into the air above you, first with one hand and then with the other. Next, first with one hand, then with the other, push down as if you were pushing something into the floor. Then push forwards with each hand in turn.

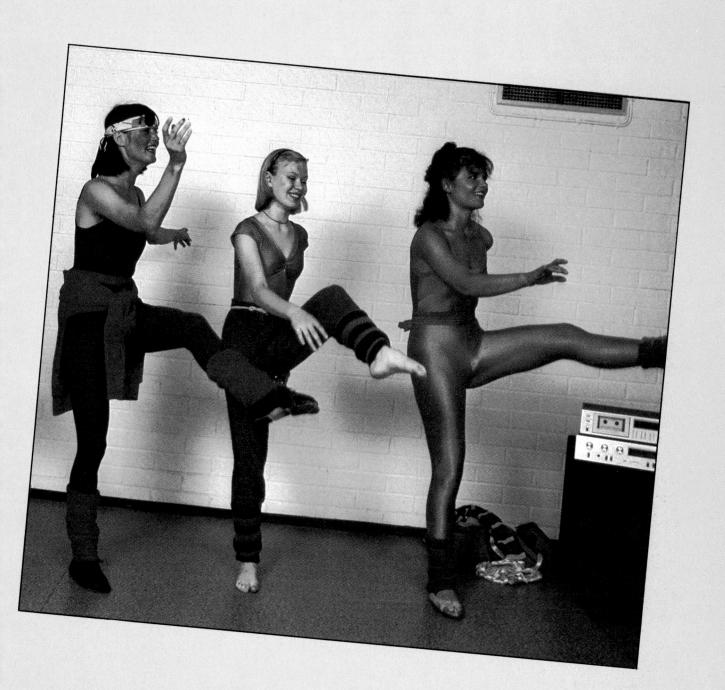

ACTIVITY

Dancing

The aim of this part of the Home Workout (which should last five minutes) is to move about vigorously, extending muscles further than before, burning up energy and mobilizing fat from your body reserves. Vigorous disco dancing is ideal, and other types of dancing are almost as good if they are done at a brisk tempo. If you like, choreograph your own routine. It is important to keep moving, so if you find yourself getting really out of breath, slow down to half tempo for a minute, then continue at the faster speed. If you want to dance but are short of ideas we give some suggestions (see panel). If dancing is not for you, do room running instead.

Room running

This section, which is an alternative to dancing, takes five minutes. It is possible to have a good run even in a small house or flat, provided you don't try to race. If you don't mind being seen by neighbours, you can include any paths outside the building; otherwise, set up a 'track' around one or more rooms, moving the odd piece of furniture if necessary. Set off at a gentle jogging pace you can keep up. If you get out of breath, slow down to a walk until you get your breath back. (You should be able to sing as you run.) If you are really short of space, run on the spot, preferably on carpet, raising your feet at least four inches off the ground.

Skipping

This section lasts two and a half minutes. Skipping is a demanding exercise which burns up two or three times as many calories per minute as jogging. It requires skill. Even people who are reasonably fit (particularly men) may find it difficult to begin with, and will have to concentrate on developing their skill. When you do become skilful at it, skipping is a superb way of building stamina (as generations of boxers have discovered). It exercises the heart and lungs as well as the legs, arms, chest and shoulders.

A skipping rope, which can be made from a sash cord or washing

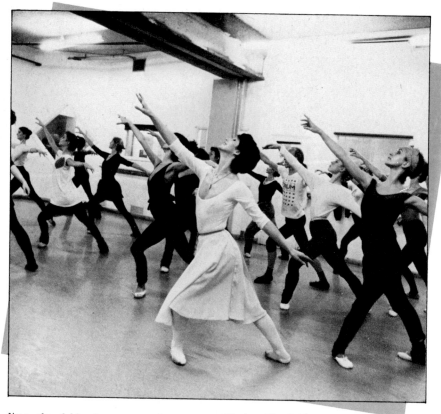

line, should be long enough to reach from one armpit to another when you are standing on it. It is advisable to skip on soft grassy ground or on carpet. If you are careful you will probably be able to skip indoors – perhaps in a passage.

Begin with the basic skipping step: feet together, weight on the balls of the feet, arms at the side, knees slightly bent. Practise about 50 skips without the rope. Then start skipping with the rope, remembering to start with it *behind* your feet, and avoiding the common mistake of jumping too soon and getting your legs tangled in the rope. If you really find skipping too difficult for any reason, do more room running instead.

Do 50 skips with the rope. You will be doing very well if you can manage this much without getting the rope tangled several times. Add 10 skips a day if you can. Try to remember any skipping rhymes from childhood ('I like coffee, I like tea ...') and recite them to help set up a good rhythm and to count the number of skips you do. Don't spend more than two and a half minutes on this section.

Stair climbing

Your aim is to walk *up* a total of about 100 steps in two and a half minutes. In practice this will probably mean going up one flight between six and 10 times. If the 100 steps take you less than two minutes, you are doing well.

If there are no stairs where you live, you can get a similar effect by stepping on and off a low stool, or, more strenuously, a chair. Alternate your leading foot. This exercise is more strenuous because there is no period of rest equivalent to going downstairs. Try to keep going for a full minute, rest and do more. If you find this too difficult do room running instead.

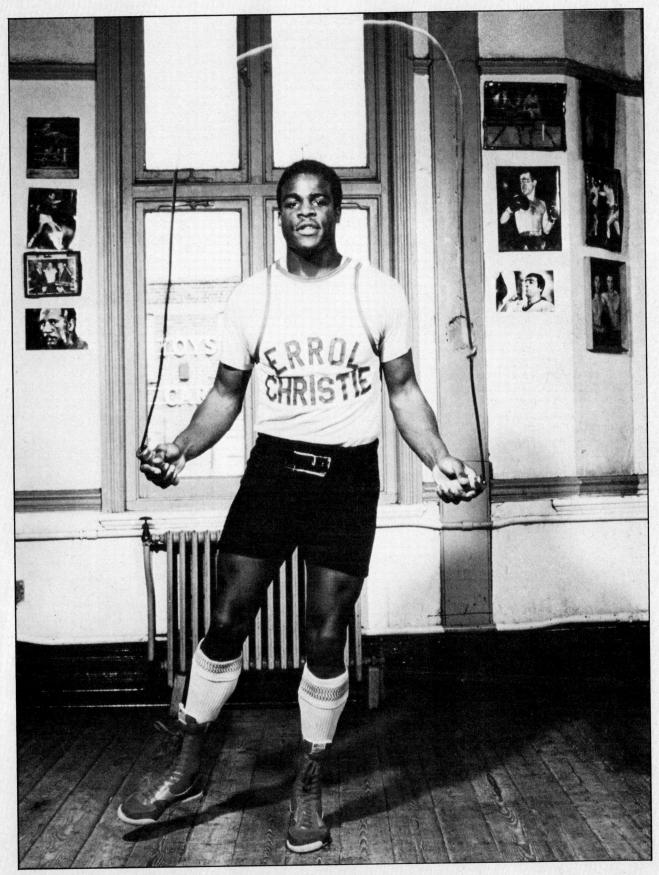

Middleweight boxer Errol Christie.

B FOR BEHAVIOUR

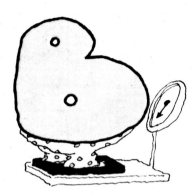

Anyone who has followed the sort of diet which offers a piece of dry toast for breakfast, an olive for lunch, and a crispbread and lettuce leaf for dinner knows how it feels to crave food so badly that after a few days your will breaks and you clear the refrigerator of whole chickens and six helpings of pudding.

Carried to extremes, bingeing – strict dieting followed by a frenzy of eating – may require professional help to untangle the web of psychological problems underlying it. But ordinary dieters, too, can benefit from understanding what causes it, and how the pattern can be changed.

Binge Eating

Portrait of a Binge Eater

She is almost certainly female because the social pressures on women to be slim are stronger than on men, although strict dieting can turn either sex to bingeing. Since her teens she has obsessively monitored her weight and shape, and compared them to an imaginary ideal inspired by advertising, fashion, other women, boyfriends, etc.

In public she eats little, and may keep to a narrow range of low calorie foods for days, or even weeks. Eventually her will breaks and, in a frenzy of guilt, she gorges herself uncontrollably. It is the feeling of helpless abandonment to food, rather than how much she eats, which sets her apart from other overeaters. For the binge-eater, a blowout is followed by such self-disgust that shortly afterwards she resolves to diet again, and the cycle of starving followed by gorging is repeated. Some even risk their health by regularly eating huge amounts then vomiting or taking laxatives.

How dieting makes you binge

Although subtle social and emotional pressures underlie chronic bingeing, biology also plays a part. If your body is starved of food for long enough, you naturally feel physically and psychologically deprived. In one US experiment in the 1940s, a group of normal healthy young men, who were conscientious objectors in the Second World War, volunteered to be given consistently less food than they needed to maintain their body weight. The aim of the experiment was to investigate effects of semi-starvation. The result was to turn the young men into binge eaters in a few weeks.

They had agreed to abide by very rigid diet rules and, like chronic dieters, they became obsessed with thoughts of food and felt mortified if they 'cheated'. Then when they were allowed to eat freely, they gorged themselves until they had re-gained all the weight they had lost, or more.

Dieting causes binge eating because to succeed dieters have to disassociate themselves from normal hunger pangs, says Dr Peter Herman, a psychologist at the university of Toronto. Whether or not you eat then depends on your emotional state, which is hard to control. He recommends what he calls 'undieting'. 'Dieting leads to bingeing, which messes up the metabolism and the natural

ARE YOU A BINGER?

Answer 'yes' or 'no' to the following questions:

- [ ] Do you often diet?
- [ ] Have you ever lost more than 20 lbs in one month?
- [ ] Have you ever gained more than 6 lbs in one week?
- [ ] Does your weight change by more than 2 lbs in a typical week?
- [ ] If you gained or lost 5 lbs would it affect your social life?
- [ ] Do you feel you give too much time and thought to food?
- [ ] After you overeat, do you feel guilty?
- [ ] Are you always aware of what you eat?
- [ ] Is the heaviest you have been more than a stone over your ideal weight?

If you answered 'yes' to more than four questions you are probably a binge-eater.

(Adapted from a questionnaire devised by Dr Peter Herman)

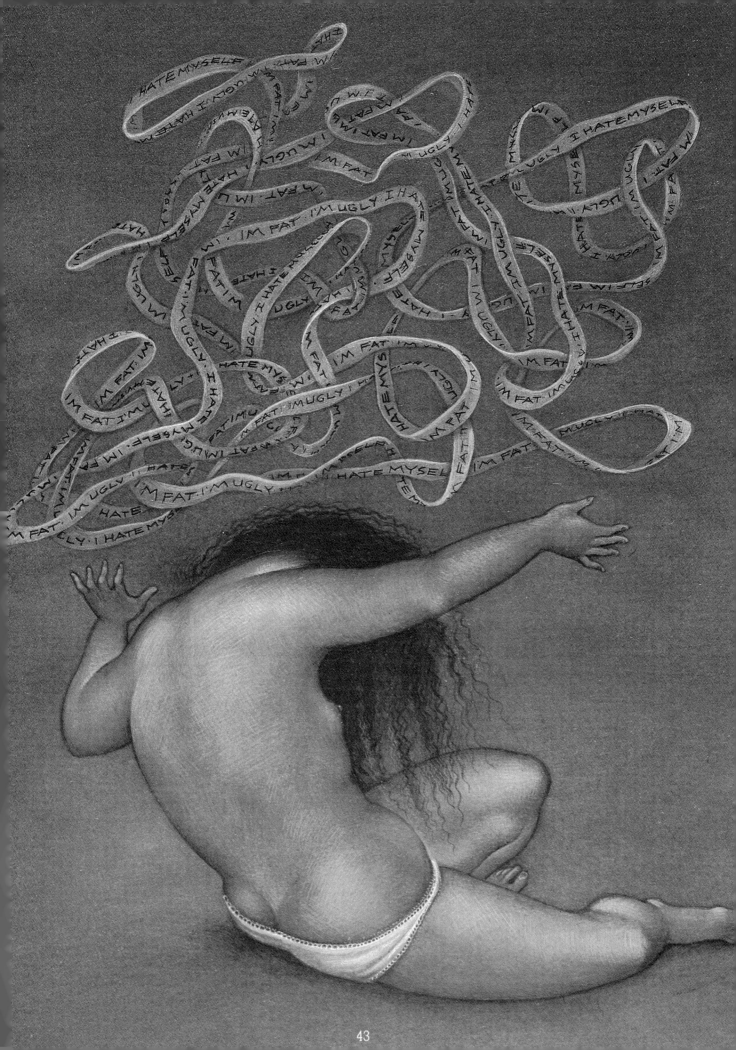

B E H A V I O U R

regulation of eating,' he says.

Dr Hubert Lacey is a psychiatrist at St George's Hospital Medical School in London who successfully treats women with *bulimia nervosa* (the bingeing-vomiting cycle) by combining group psychotherapy with behaviour modification. Thirty of his patients (all women) kept a record of their moods and food intake. They agreed to stop slimming during the 10-week programme, to eat a set amount of carbohydrate, and to meet as a group. At the end of the programme, 28 had stopped bingeing and vomiting. Two years later they were still eating normally.

They were extreme cases, but the principles of their treatment can be applied to less severe bingeing behaviour, as in the plan that follows.

A six-point plan to beat bingeing

1. Stop trying to restrict your food intake (at least for now). Continual strict dieting unbalances your metabolism, distorts your appetite control, starves your body of nutrients and feeds your guilt. You can still follow the Constant Energy Diet because it does not involve denying yourself food.
2. Eat three meals a day to stave off temptation and to bring order to erratic eating habits. Rediscover breakfast and never miss a meal, especially after you have been bingeing.
3. Reconsider your attitudes to everyday problems.
Don't delay: if you are putting off all sorts of things until you are slimmer, your expectations of what life will be like at your 'ideal' weight are probably unrealistic. Start doing them now instead of using weight as an excuse.

Avoid extremism: bingers see things in black and white, with no shades of grey. They judge themselves and others almost solely on the basis of size, and brand themselves total failures because they do not conform to arbitrary standards. They are either 'on' or 'off' a diet and are prone to reason that if they have eaten two biscuits they might as well finish the packet. In

experiments disguised as taste tests binge-eaters ate more ice-cream if they had already had a milk shake which they thought was high in calories than if they had had nothing beforehand. And they ate still more if they had had two milk shakes.

Take control: binge eaters tend to over-react to bad moods and ordinary daily crises. They may also be unassertive and have trouble structuring their lives. Acquiring a sense of mastery over everyday life helps to break the bingeing habit.
4. Take regular vigorous exercise, following one of the programmes in this book. Exercise helps weight loss without dieting, eases stress and depression, improves body image and gives a feeling of taking control over your life.
5. When you have gained some stability over your eating, start to allow yourself 'forbidden' foods. The only way to stop fearing foods such as bread, cake, cheese or chocolate, or whatever it is you don't normally allow yourself when dieting, is to give yourself permission to eat them. Learn to eat them in moderation and without feeling anxious. Taking the guilt out of eating is part of all successful approaches to bingeing. For instance, Susie Orbach, author of *Fat is a Feminist Issue*, tells compulsive eaters to stock their kitchen with taboo foods; Dr Roy Fitzgerald, a Philadelphia psychiatrist, organizes annual chocolate-weekends to take the anxiety out of chocolate eating, and Dr William Freemouw, a psychologist at the University of West Virginia, gets binge-eaters to eat a small amount of their problem food in front of him and won't let them leave until they feel happy about it.
6. If, after following the positive advice in our eating plan, you're still obsessed with food, abandon dieting for good and follow only the Activity and Behaviour programmes. Many reformed binge-eaters find that, once they start to eat normally they lose weight slowly without dieting and stabilise at a weight a little higher than they once aimed for. Taking more exercise should reduce your weight anyway without dieting.

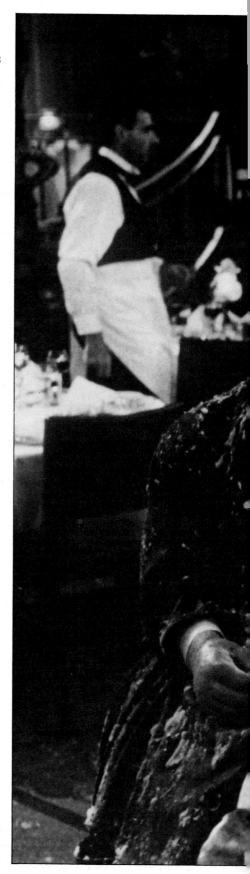

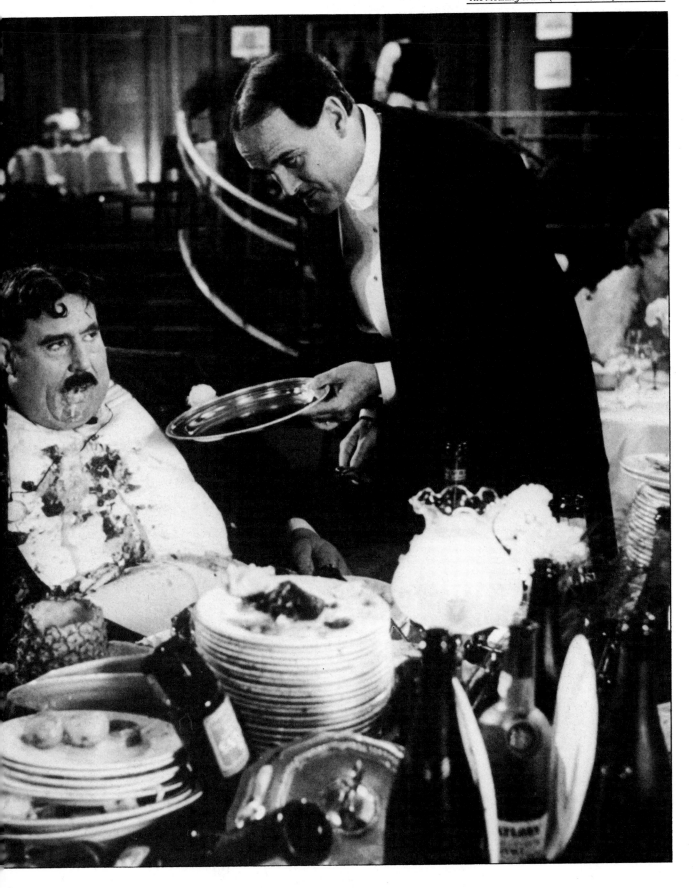

C FOR CONSUMPTION

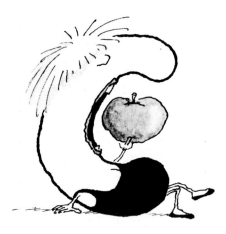

A shortage of fibre in your diet could be one reason why you are overweight. Until about 10 years ago only a minority of vegetarians and health food fanatics believed that fibre was important for good health. Doctors and nutritionists generally believed that it was of no value. For years they had been telling people with digestive problems to go on bland diets without fibre; now it is widely accepted that such advice was mistaken, that dietary fibre is important for everyone, and particularly for people who are overweight... so, more bulk, less hulk.

Fibre

The general attitude to fibre changed when two campaigning doctors, Dennis Burkitt and Hugh Trowell, who had both been medical missionaries in Africa, published their research. They had been struck by the number of Western diseases which were virtually unknown among Africans eating traditional foods. Among the diseases investigated by Burkitt and Trowell were several diseases of the bowel common in the West, such as appendicitis, diverticulitis, piles and cancer of the bowel, as well as gallstones, diabetes, varicose veins and heart disease. All these diseases were rare among Africans living traditionally, and Burkitt and Trowell argued that too much sugar and too little fibre in the diet were the cause.

In Europe obesity and diabetes emerged as common conditions among the upper classes in the late 18th century, when refined flour and sugar began to be consumed in quantity by wealthy people. Now that everyone can afford as much sugar and refined food as they wish, people who are overweight are found in all social classes. Similarly, Africans who live in cities and eat a European diet are often grossly overweight. Yet obesity was rare among Africans at the beginning of the 20th century, when the continent was being opened up to European influence and trade, and is still rare among Africans and other people who eat a traditional diet of unprocessed seeds, vegetables and fruit, which contain a lot of dietary fibre.

Dr Roland Weinsier, of the University of Alabama School of Medicine, has shown that fewer calories are consumed on a high-fibre diet. He gave a group of people a high-bulk diet for five days and a low-bulk diet – potato crisps, hot dogs and a lot of meat – for another five days. The low-bulk diet was twice as concentrated as the high bulk diet, yet when the volunteers were allowed to eat as much as they liked of each diet it was found that they ate almost twice as many calories when on the low-bulk diet – suggesting that bulk has an important effect on how much people eat.

The bulky wholefood diet took longer to chew – 69 minutes per day instead of 52 for the low-bulk diet. Surprisingly, the volunteers showed no preference for one diet over the other. Weinsier suggests that the sheer volume of the high-bulk diet induces a feeling of fullness and satisfaction even though fewer calories have been consumed. In addition, bulky food is digested more slowly and so keeps the blood sugar level steady.

The Constant Energy Diet (discussed more fully in Week Three) aims to introduce you to a more natural, healthy and enjoyable way of eating which includes more fibre. Fibre is useful for slimmers because it fills up the stomach and bowel, giving a feeling of satisfaction. Fibre has a beneficial laxative effect – most of the fibre remains undigested and so forms a soft, bulky stool which passes quickly through the body. At the same time the bulkiness of the stool means that about two per cent of the food (measured in calories) passes through the bowel without being absorbed.

Adding fibre to your diet will certainly help you to slim, but it is also necessary to reduce the amount of refined foods such as sugar and white flour in your food intake. Some people do not realise this, and make the mistake of eating sweet biscuits with fibre added in the form of bran. Such products may be preferable to the same product without bran, but the added bran is not sufficient to counteract the extra calories from sugar and fat. Furthermore, added bran is not the most suitable form of fibre for slimmers, and, if taken in quantity on a reducing diet, there is some risk of its causing mild malnutrition. Added bran is not recommended on the Constant Energy Diet. Fibre is provided naturally in the diet by the inclusion of vegetables, fruit (see An Apple a Day ... But Two Are Better) and rice.

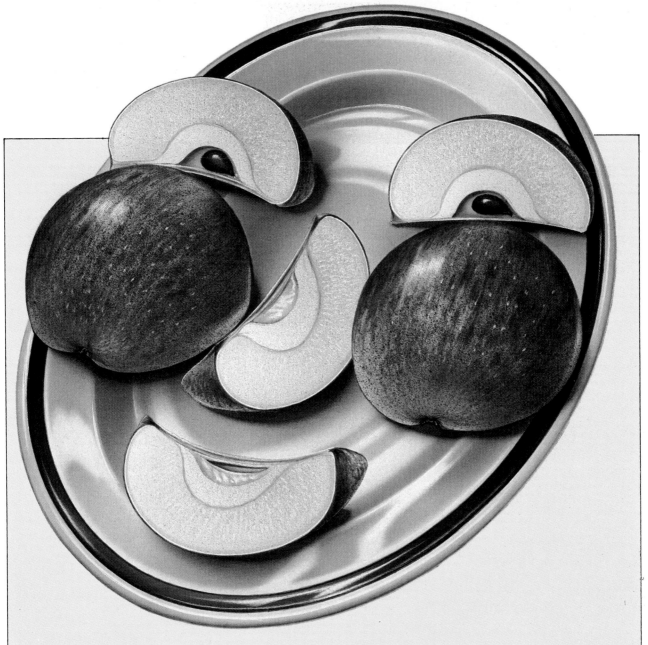

AN APPLE A DAY ... BUT TWO ARE BETTER

Generations of people have believed that an apple a day brings good health. One apple may be sufficient but two are even better for the slimmer. This is because apples contain plenty of fibre and are digested slowly, releasing their sugar steadily to keep the blood sugar topped up. Apples need no preparation, most people like them, and so they make a very convenient natural snack. Try and include two raw apples in your diet every day; the purpose of the apple snack is to provide a constant supply of energy which can be particularly useful between meals.

Apples have long been recommended in weight reducing diets, but their importance as a 'slow food', which releases energy slowly and steadily, has only recently been understood. The main source of energy in apples, as in most fruit, is fructose (fruit sugar) and so apples are excellent for people who crave something sweet. Fructose is absorbed into the body and broken down to glucose (the sugar in blood) more slowly than other sugars and so provides longer lasting energy.

An experiment done by Dr Kenneth Heaton and colleagues at Bristol University demonstrated dramatically how much more satisfying raw apples are than apple juice or apple purée. Heaton gave 10 volunteers either whole Golden Delicious apples, or the same amount of apple made into purée or juice. It took the volunteers an average of 17 minutes to eat the apples, six minutes to consume the purée and only one and a half minutes to drink the juice. The volunteers reported that the whole apples were more satisfying. Blood sugar rose after all the different forms of apple. But, after the apple juice, insulin in the blood rose to twice the level that it did after the consumption of whole apples. About two hours later blood sugar was back to normal after the whole apples but, after the juice, it plummetted to below normal – to a level usually associated with hunger.

Apples, like most fruit, are about 85% water. This gives apples an important advantage over bran; an apple is immediately filling and easier and more satisfying to chew. A small apple weighing about four and a half ounces only provides about 40 calories and is also a good source of filling fibre (about 4 grams). Apple is much preferable to bran as a source of fibre because it does not contain the phytate found in bran which in excess can lead to a deficiency of minerals in the diet. Furthermore the fibre in apples, pectin, has the beneficial effect for the heart of lowering the amount of cholesterol in the blood – an effect not produced by bran. Apples are also a good source of minerals and of several vitamins, particularly carotene, which is converted into vitamin A and is good for the skin.

CONSUMPTION

Rice

Rice is good for slimmers. It is filling, and, like other grains, it is not digested too rapidly, so it keeps the blood sugar topped up and hunger at bay. Along with bread and potatoes, rice is often avoided by slimmers quite unnecessarily. Rice is an integral part of most of the dishes that follow, which are designed to help slimmers who in the past have tended to shun carbohydrates.

Brown rice, which contains more fibre and more vitamins than white, is the ideal choice for the slimmer. But white rice, which is easier to cook and more widely appreciated, is also digested quite slowly and provides steady energy. The Constant Energy Diet is designed to be enjoyed by family and friends, so all these dishes may be cooked with white rice if you prefer.

Recipes

Portion size

Our recipes have been calculated to be about the right quantity for a family of four: two parents and two children under 10. However, it is not possible for us to tell you exactly what quantities to cook because the amount you and your companions eat will depend so much on how active you are. Age and size are also important – young people and large people need more food than older or smaller people. A family with two teenage boys would probably need to cook larger quantities. The Constant Energy Diet is not a calorie controlled diet; you have to be guided in the amount you cook and eat by appetite. The ABC Bodyplan aims at developing your knowlege of the right foods to eat and insight into your eating habits so that you learn to control your appetite naturally. That is why we only give you general advice here.

In working out these recipes we have calculated on four ounces of meat without bone, five ounces of chicken without bone, or five ounces of fish, per person. From the strictly nutritional point of view, three ounces of meat or fish provides more than enough protein for most adults. We chose these quantities so that the recipes would be acceptable to people who may have been used to eating very little starchy food. However, the quantities may be altered to reduce the meat or fish portion to three ounces per person and to increase the vegetable and carbohydrate portion accordingly.

Lemon Chicken with Rice And Leeks

One 3-3½ lb (1.5kg) chicken, neatly tied with string; 1½ lb (675g) leeks, chopped; 4 carrots, chopped; 8oz (225g) rice; 2tbsp olive or sunflower oil; salt and pepper; 8 sprigs parsley; about 3½ pints (2.1 litres) stock.for the sauce: 2 egg yolks; 2tbsp lemon juice.

Use an oval fireproof casserole to cook this in if possible: if not a round pan will do. Heat the oil in the pan over a medium heat, put in the chicken and brown it on all sides until golden. Remove the chicken and put in the carrots. Stir them around for 2-3 minutes until they are glossy and just beginning to colour. Return the chicken to the pan and pour on the warm stock to cover the thighs of the bird. Bring gently to the boil, skim, and add salt, pepper and 4 sprigs of parsley tied together. Cover the casserole and put it in a warm 300°F (150°C, gas mark 2) oven for 40-45 minutes. Check that the carrots are tender, but not too soft. With a slotted spoon, remove them to a serving dish and keep warm. Put the rice and leeks into the casserole and continue to cook in the oven for a further 20 minutes.

Meanwhile beat the egg yolks in a bowl, adding the lemon juice a little at a time. When the rice is cooked the chicken should also be done. Remove the chicken and leave to rest in a warm place. Drain the rice and leeks, reserving the stock, and put them with the carrots in the serving dish. Put the egg and lemon juice into a double boiler and gradually add ¼ pint (150ml) of the chicken stock. Heat gently, stirring all the time, until the sauce thickens.

Carve the chicken and serve with a portion of rice sprinkled with some chopped parsley and some vegetables. Serve the sauce separately. This amount should make a good hearty meal for 4, leaving quite a lot of chicken for another meal and enough stock to make some good soup.

Rice, Spinach and Nuts

8oz (225g) rice; 1 pint (600ml) stock; 1½ lb (675g) fresh spinach, or 12oz (350g) frozen spinach; 2oz (50g) walnut pieces; 4oz (100-125g) cheddar cheese, grated; 1 lemon, juice only; salt and pepper; 2oz (50g) brown breadcrumbs (optional); parsley, finely chopped (optional).

Cook the rice in the stock with a lid on the pan. The rice should be done in approximately 15 minutes, by which time the liquid should be absorbed. If not, put it over a high heat for a few moments. Wash and cook the spinach, adding no liquid but that which clings to the leaves. (Cook frozen spinach according to the directions on the packet.) When it is soft, drain it in a sieve, pressing out as much liquid as possible. Put the spinach on a board and chop it finely. Mix together the spinach, rice, walnut pieces and cheese, add the lemon juice and season to taste.

Either serve this as it is straight from the pan, or put the spinach and rice into an ovenproof dish and cover with the breadcrumbs mixed with chopped parsley. Cook in a moderate oven 350°F (180°C, gas mark 4), for 20 minutes or until the top is nicely browned. This is a very quick and easy dish to make and it also reheats well. Start the meal with some soup and have brown bread and butter on the table.

Rice and Lentil Salad

4oz (100-125g) rice; 4oz (100-125g) brown or green lentils; 4 tomatoes, peeled and chopped; 1 bunch spring onions, chopped; 1 small bunch coriander, washed and chopped; 5oz (150g) yoghurt; ½ lemon, juice only; salt and pepper.

Cook the rice and lentils separately. Drain, mix together and allow to cool. Stir in the tomatoes, spring onions, coriander and the yoghurt mixed with the lemon juice. Season with salt and pepper and serve.

If fresh coriander is unavailable, use a dessertspoonful of coriander seeds instead. Roast them in a hot, dry frying pan and crush them with a pestle and mortar. The taste will be different, but just as delicious.

Stuffed Lettuce Leaves

1 large cos or Webb's lettuce; 6oz (175g) rice; 2tbsp olive or sunflower oil; 2 small onions; 3oz (75g) celery, chopped; 4oz (100-125g) tomatoes, peeled and chopped; 1½oz (40g) pinenuts; 1½oz (40g) raisins; 6oz (175g) ham, cut in ½in (1cm) pieces; salt and pepper; 1tsp allspice; ½ pint (300ml) tomato juice; juice of 1 lemon.

Cook the rice in boiling salted water, and drain well. Cook the onions and celery slowly in the oil in a heavy pan until soft but not coloured. Stir in the tomatoes, pinenuts, raisins and ham, and season with salt, pepper and allspice.

Put the lettuce in a suitable container, cover with boiling water and leave to stand for 2 minutes. Drain well and separate the leaves, rinsing off any dirt with cold water. Place a tablespoonful of the mixture near the base of each lettuce leaf. Fold the bottom of the leaf over the mixture, fold the two sides into the middle, then roll up.

Place the little parcels side by side in a large oiled pan with the loose ends of the leaves underneath. Pack as many of the parcels into the pan as possible (you may have to cook them in two batches). Pour the tomato and lemon juice into the pan together with ½ pint (300ml) of water. Cover the pan with a plate which will slip down inside and keep the parcels from unrolling, and cook slowly for about 30 minutes. Remove the parcels to a warmed dish, and serve the remaining juice as a sauce, reducing it quickly if it is too liquid.

Paella

Serves 6-8

8oz (225g) firm white fish (turbot, halibut or cod); 8oz (225g) prawns in their shells; 12 mussels, in their shells, cleaned; 2tbsp olive or sunflower oil; 2 medium onions, sliced; 12oz (350g) rice, Italian risotto or arborio if possible; 2 red or yellow peppers, seeded and chopped; 1 clove of garlic, crushed; 8oz (225g) green beans, fresh or frozen; 1 packet of saffron or 1tsp paprika; 1 bay leaf; salt and pepper; 8oz (225g) small squid (optional).

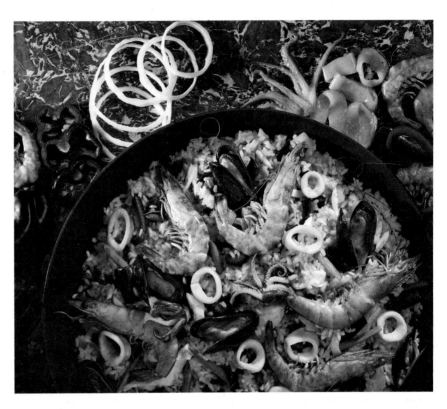

Heat the oil in a large heavy frying pan and cook the onions and the peppers until limp. Add the rice and the crushed garlic to the pan and stir until the rice is glossy. Remove from the heat.

Poach the white fish in a pan with enough water to cover, adding salt and pepper and a bay leaf. The time for the cooking will be determined by the thickness of the fish and not by its weight. Cook it very slowly, with the surface of the water barely moving, for approximately 10-15 minutes, testing to see if the fish is cooked. Remove it from the pan and keep in a warm place. If using squid, poach in the same water until tender.

Measure 1½ pints (900ml) of stock into the pan with the rice, peppers and onions, and add the saffron or paprika. Return to the heat, bring to the boil and simmer gently, stirring from time to time. Put the prawns with the fish in a warm place. Cook the beans until just tender and keep hot. Put the mussels in a pan over a medium heat until the shells open. Keep them with the other fish, straining their liquid into the paella. As the rice is cooked the liquid should all be absorbed and evaporated. If this is not the case increase the heat and allow the rice to dry off. Stir in the flaked fish and squid and arrange the mussels and shrimps in their shells round the edge of the pan, or remove them from their shells and stir them into the paella.

YOUR ABC DIARY: Week Two					Starting date:			
	WALKING		JOGGING/ WALKING		SWIMMING		HOME WORKOUT	OTHER EXERCISE (e.g. cycling)
	Mins	Miles*	Mins	Miles*	Mins	Lengths	Mins	Mins
Monday								
Tuesday								
Wednesday								
Thursday								
Friday								
Saturday								
Sunday								
TOTAL								

* approximate distance, optional

ABC ROAD TEST		mins		mph				
BODY MEASUREMENTS	Date / /	Chest	Waist	Hips	Arms	Legs	Weight	

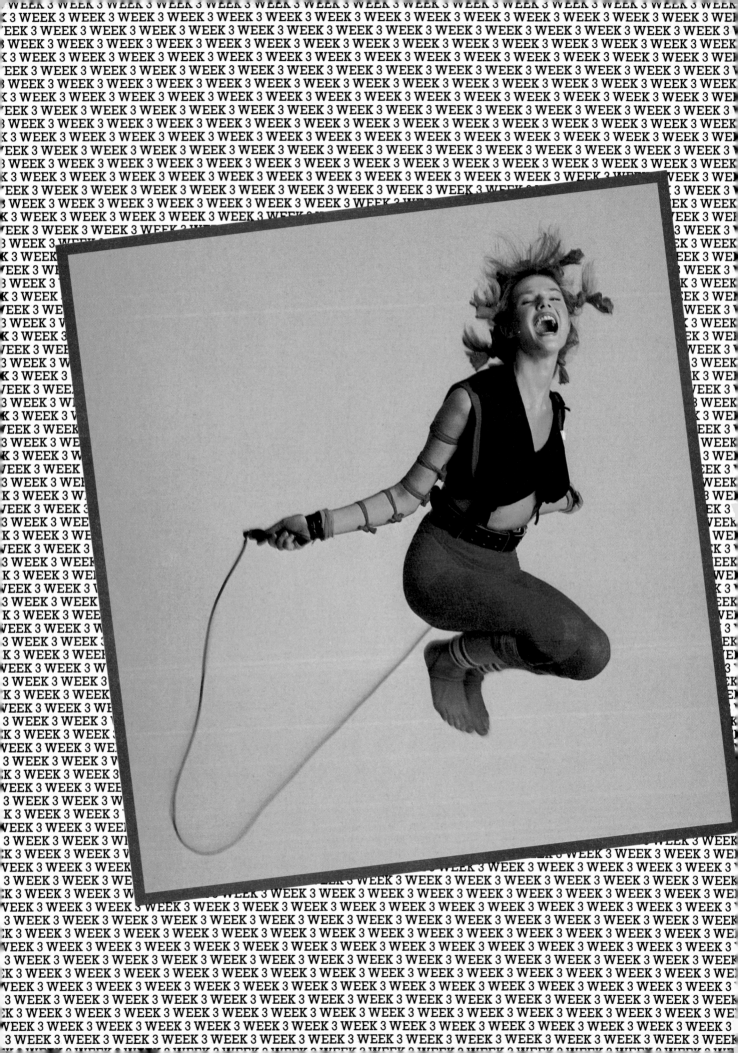

Week 3

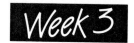

Week 3

A FOR ACTIVITY

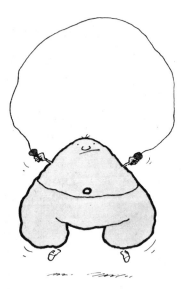

The way that muscles strengthen is through a process of slight injury and repair. To allow sufficient time for this repair and healing, it is a good idea to vary your activities, so that you are not repeatedly putting strain on the same muscles, especially if you are over 35. This week we make suggestions for new activities, such as cycling, dancing and sports to play in the garden, which you can include in your schedule for variety. Set aside time for five exercise sessions of 30 to 40 minutes, vary your activities from day to day, and incorporate more than one activity in a single session, if you like, so long as you keep moving. If you are walking or jogging, try to increase your speed and to find interesting or scenic routes so far as possible. Remember to attempt the ABC Road Test once a week as a measure of how well you are doing.

Do five exercise sessions this week.

Walking Programme

At least four of your five exercise sessions should be spent walking. Non-walking sessions should be used for games or dancing which are at least as demanding in energy. If these alternative sessions are less energetic than walking then you should spend a longer time doing them. In any case, aim to increase each walking session to 40 minutes if you can do this without overtiring yourself.

Jogging Programme

Jogging 1
- Walk briskly for five minutes.
- Jog for one minute then walk for one minute. Do this 10 times.
- Walk for 15 minutes with short jogs if you want to.
  Total exercise time: 40 minutes
- Finish with the Cool Down Stretches (see Week One).

You are now attempting to increase your time from approximately 30 to 40 minutes in order to burn fat more effectively. If this is too difficult, or the sessions too tiring, stick to your previous programme for another week.

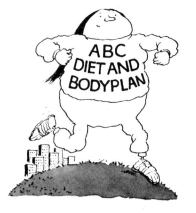

Jogging 2
- Walk briskly for five minutes.
- Jog for three minutes, then walk for two minutes. Do this five or six times.
- Walk for 10 minutes or so.
  Total exercise time: 40 minutes
- Finish with the Cool Down Stretches (see Week One).

You are still building up the length and intensity of exercise, so expect to feel tired and to need more sleep.

Swimming Programme

Swimming 1
Warm-up
- Use this warm-up period to practise any strokes you are unsure of or to do the Pool Exercises.

Exercise
- Swim 12 lengths, alternating your best stroke with one other stroke, resting between lengths if you wish. For a more vigorous workout, swim without resting or use sidestroke or backstroke, so that you can work harder without breathing problems.
- End with the Pool Exercises (see Week One).

Swimming 2
You should be able to do two strokes other than side stroke and basic backstroke to follow this plan. Whichever these strokes are (for instance, breaststroke and crawl, or crawl and full backstroke), we refer to them as your first and second strokes.

Warm-up
- Do two lengths of your first stroke, one length of your second stroke and one length of your first stroke. Then repeat, to make a total of eight lengths. Rest between lengths if you need to.

Exercise
- Do six lengths, alternating your first stroke with basic or full backstroke.
- Do four lengths, alternating your second stroke with sidestroke or another stroke.
- Do two lengths of any stroke.
  Total: 20 lengths
- End with the Pool Exercises (optional).

The Home Workout

1. Warm Up Exercises (see Week Two) – five minutes
2. Dancing or room running – five minutes
3. Skipping – two and a half minutes
4. Stair climbing – two and a half minutes
5. Repeat steps 1 to 4
Total exercise time: 30 minutes.
6. Do the Cool Down Stretches (see Week One).

Dancing or room running

Experiment with new dance moves, but keep them energetic. If you prefer, spend five minutes dancing and five room running.

Skipping

This week the aim is to learn the skipping two-step, which is basically jogging as you skip, but bringing the knees up. For those to whom this manoeuvre is not obvious, here's how to do it: start by jumping with feet together. After a few jumps raise one foot a little in front and hop 10 times on the other. Switch feet and repeat. When you have mastered this, raise alternate feet to get a jogging action, lifting the knees. Aim to do 100 of these skips in two and a half minutes, and increase the number by 10 a day.

If you cannot manage 100 skips in the time, don't worry. You just need more practice.

Stair climbing

Last week the target was to walk *up* 100 steps in two and a half minutes. From now on, aim to build up steadily until you can get *up* 200 steps in that time, which means taking them at a steady run. Meanwhile work at a speed you find challenging and increase it when you can.

Stool-stepping: Do as many steps as you can until you are out of breath. Try to develop a steady pace which you can keep up for two and a half minutes. If this is too difficult, use a lower step until you can manage the full two and a half minutes.

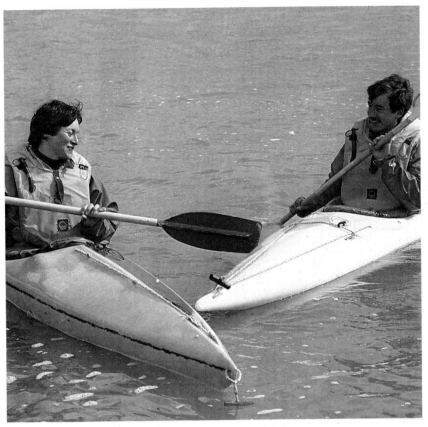

Take up Another Activity

After two weeks of preparation many people will be ready to add on another activity which provides extra interest as well as exercise. Begin by replacing one of your five weekly exercise sessions, if you want to, with some other activity. Continue with at least four sessions a week of walking, jogging, swimming or Home Workout, because you can monitor your progress accurately in these sessions and so demand more of yourself.

Squash is one of the best sports for burning energy and inducing fat loss, but it is too strenuous for many people at this stage. You should start with cycling, dancing, golf, table tennis, tennis, or badminton. They will help you to lose weight as you gain in fitness and proficiency.

If you want to include tennis or badminton in your schedule, it is best not to play formal games unless you are very proficient and have a well matched partner. Simply aim to keep the ball or shuttlecock in play as long as possible, and when you fail to hit it, run – don't walk – to pick it up. Otherwise, you spend most of the time just standing around the court.

You can buy a cheap badminton or soft tennis kit at most sports shops for under £20. Rig up the net anywhere there is enough space and have fun for an hour or so hitting the ball or shuttlecock around. An hour may be roughly equivalent to half an hour's organized exercise in one of our plans. Another fun sport is swing-ball, which again can be bought in most sports shops, although it may be a bit more expensive. Swing-ball takes up very little space – most city gardens are big enough – is energetic and can be played alone or with a partner.

Because dancing is so enjoyable, many people do not think of it as exercise. Yet it generally involves much more muscular movement and exertion than walking. It doesn't matter which type you choose.

ACTIVITY

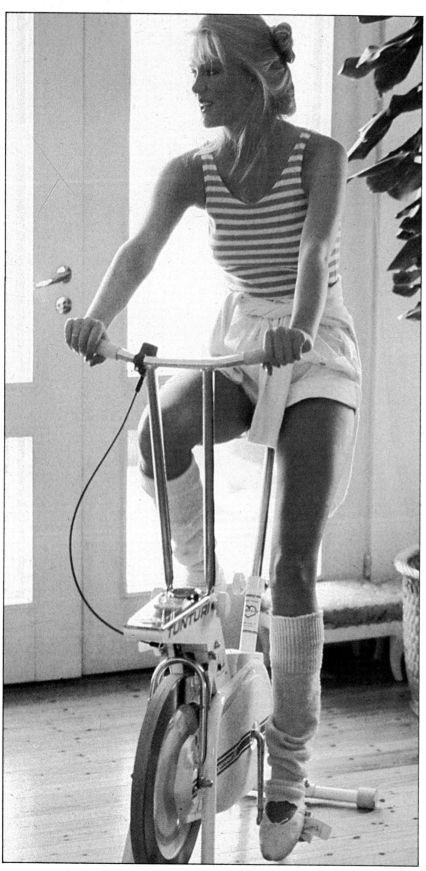

Cycling

Cycling is an excellent form of exercise and can use up a lot of calories. The further or faster you cycle the more calories you use.

Taking a six mile journey as an example: 20 minutes would be a very good time and 35 minutes would be slow. The total amount of calories burnt up is roughly the same whatever the time taken.

A journey of between five and 10 miles per day is a reasonable distance to cycle. A fast 20 minute ride to work in the morning and back in the evening can be counted as equivalent to a fast 30 minute ride once a day.

Once you have established cycling as a routine you should measure out your regular journeys on the map and time them. Aim gradually to demand more of yourself by doing longer, faster or more frequent journeys. Cycling at 10 miles an hour is the equivalent of a sedate walk if conditions are good; 20 miles an hour is the equivalent of a good run. A heavy bicycle, heavy luggage, traffic, adverse wind, hills and poor surfaces will all slow you down. So 10mph may be a fair speed for the bicycle commuter with a heavy bag.

If you feel any pain or discomfort in your knees, alternate cycling with another activity so as to give joints and tissues a chance to rest.

Exercise bicycles

Exercise bicycles are also a good way of working off calories. But they are expensive and you might find stationary cycling boring after a while – although you can watch TV or listen to music while doing it. It isn't worth buying a cheap bike. They are not comfortable to ride because the resistance is worked by screwing a pad on to the wheel. The best ones have a heavy flywheel which is restrained by a belt operated by an adjustable lever.

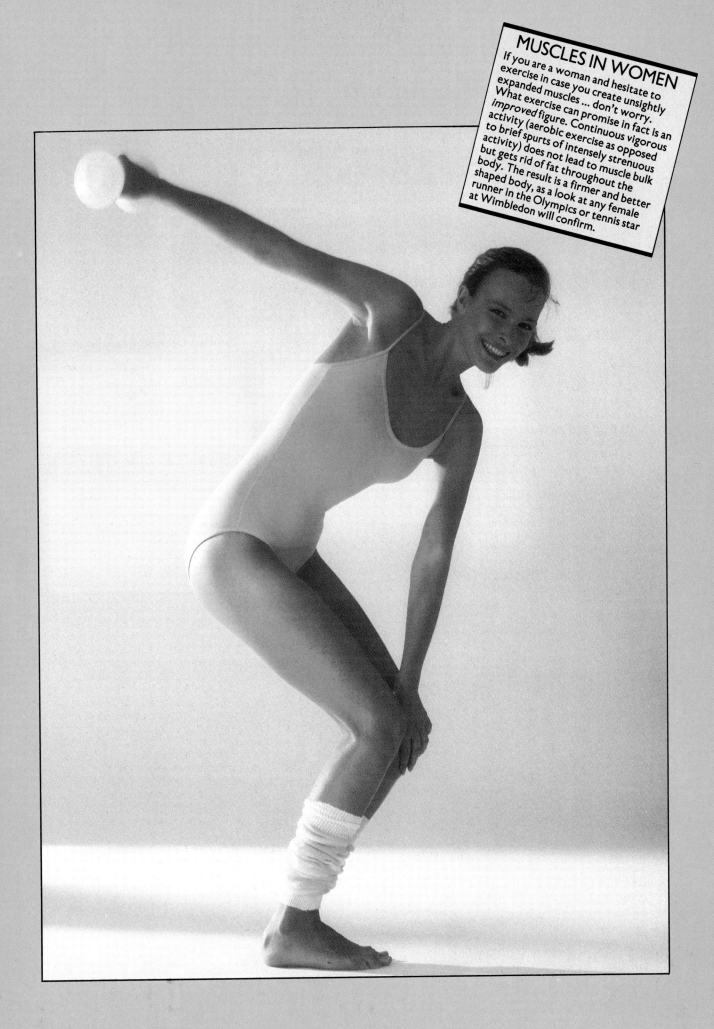

MUSCLES IN WOMEN

If you are a woman and hesitate to exercise in case you create unsightly expanded muscles ... don't worry. What exercise can promise in fact is an improved figure. Continuous vigorous activity (aerobic exercise as opposed to brief spurts of intensely strenuous activity) does not lead to muscle bulk but gets rid of fat throughout the body. The result is a firmer and better shaped body, as a look at any female runner in the Olympics or tennis star at Wimbledon will confirm.

B FOR BEHAVIOUR

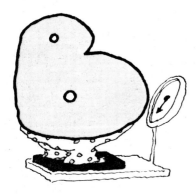

As if being overweight weren't enough, fat people have been made to feel guilty not only about what they eat but also about how they eat it. Studies of fat people's eating habits have, until recently, suggested that they are greedy, weak-willed and somehow guilty of moral torpor. They eat faster than they should, said the psychologists. They go on eating after they're full, they eat while they watch television, they're too easily tempted by the sight and smell of food and they don't chew it properly.

At the Table

Now research has shown that there are no real differences in the ways fat people and thin people eat. Whether observed in laboratory taste tests or spied upon in restaurants, fat people have been found to eat no more, and no faster, than their thin peers. They're no more likely than anyone else to eat when they're not really hungry, or to be tempted by sight and smell to scoff their food. Compulsive eaters and chronic dieters are a different matter: they have distorted their natural eating impulses by continually depriving themselves.

Nevertheless, there are good reasons for paying attention to your eating habits so that you learn to make eating a conscious choice rather than an unthinking habit. It's too easy to eat a whole meal and hardly taste it because your attention is on other things, or to munch handfuls of nuts unthinkingly over drinks, or pick at leftovers on the table as you chat over coffee.

The suggestions below are not intended to be followed slavishly. They are designed to enhance your enjoyment of food by asking you to make eating a deliberate act to which you give wholehearted attention, and they've been shown by experience to help people lose weight.

■ *Keep eating separate from other activities.* Don't read, watch TV or chat on the telephone while you're eating. Talking to companions who are eating with you is fine, but keep an eye on what you're eating.

■ *Eat in a leisurely way, sitting down,* even if it's only a snack.
■ *Don't skip meals.* If you miss a meal, you're much more likely to binge; in fact bingeing is a natural reaction to deprivation.
■ *Relax for a few seconds before starting to eat.* Take a deep breath then let the air out slowly, emptying your lungs completely.
■ *Put down utensils between mouthfuls.* This habit will seem unnatural at first but it reduces the pressure to eat fast that comes from having knife and fork poised for the next mouthful. It becomes easier to chew food more thoroughly.
■ *Leave a mouthful of each food on your plate.* The aim is not to eat less but to gain a sense of control over your eating. This is particularly important if you have a tendency to eat compulsively. It is psychologically valuable to learn how to refuse food, because it means you are no longer a victim of your own impulses or persuasion from others.
■ *Minimize temptations.* As you exercise more and learn to listen to your body more, you will get better at distinguishing true from false appetite. In the meantime, avoid making the task harder than it need be. At home, serve food on plates rather then putting dishes on the table for everyone to help themselves. That way, eating another helping involves deliberate choice. Clear plates away as soon as the course is finished. In restaurants, it is unwise to sit down in front of a basket of bread and a plate of butter if there's a 15-minute wait for food ahead. Decide what you want, put it on your plate and move the rest to another table or ask for it to be taken away.

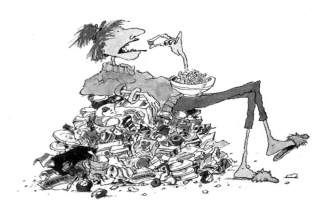

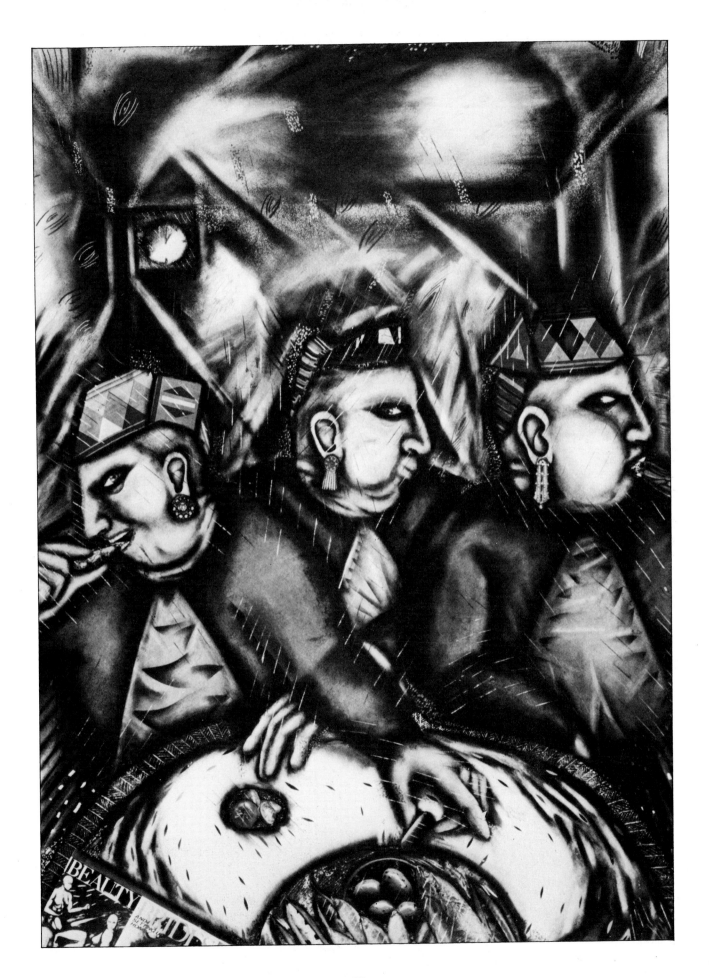

C FOR CONSUMPTION

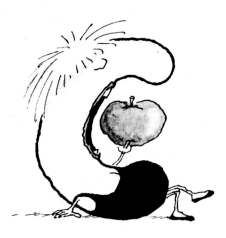

Slow food fills the energy gap and helps the body to shed fat. The Constant Energy Diet makes use of this new concept of energy balance to help people lose weight without feeling hungry, tired or unwell. It is designed to give you lasting energy throughout the day, and enough energy to take the exercise which is an essential part of the ABC Bodyplan. It builds on the steps you have already taken in Weeks One and Two to reduce the sugar content of your diet and to increase your fibre intake. The diet, together with the exercise plan, aims to produce a natural regulation of appetite, so you will not be asked to count calories or weigh food.

The Constant Energy Diet is based on research which shows how blood sugar – the body's fuel – can be kept within regular limits to make you more energetic as well as slimmer. There have been slimming diets before which promised to provide more energy but this is the first one to be based on a detailed understanding of the way different foods alter blood sugar rather than on guesswork.

Jane Furniss

Jane Furniss, 23, is the 1984 National Cross Country Champion and she has to eat a lot of food to keep going. Jane eats between 3,000 and 3,500 calories a day – twice what a lot of girls of her age eat – yet she does not carry an ounce of extra fat.

Jane, who lives at home with her parents in Sheffield, surprised many people by reaching the final of the 3,000 metres and finishing seventh in the World Championships last summer. She has now given up her job as a dental nurse to concentrate full time on running.

"I have my first training session of the day, a five-mile run, before breakfast, then come back to cornflakes, All Bran, a glass of orange juice, a cup of tea and three or four slices of toast and marmalade.

"At mid-morning I have a cup of coffee and some biscuits, but I stopped taking sugar in tea or coffee when I trained as a dental nurse and found out what it did to your teeth!

"My lunch would normally be a bowl of soup, some egg sandwiches or perhaps an egg on toast, and I try to eat plenty of fruit: usually an apple or orange after lunch.

"During the afternoon I'll have a cup of tea and some more biscuits, or perhaps a Mars bar, then at 4.30pm I do my second training session. It might be another long run, or a series of shorter, faster efforts, like 24 repetitions of 100 metres with a 100-metre recovery jog in between, or four times 600 metres. As the summer progresses, so the quantity of training decreases, but the quality improves, ready for the track season.

"In any case, when I come back, I'm usually ravenous again. I'll have my main meal of the day then: steak, or chicken, always with potatoes and vegetables, like cabbage, sprouts and carrots, with a rice pudding as a sweet. Then I have a cup of tea and biscuits, or a piece of cake. My Mum and I both love fresh cream cakes, so sometimes we treat ourselves.

"During the evening I'll have some more fruit, a banana or some grapes, and around 8pm I often drink a bottle of Guinness. My Irish coach, Jim Madigan, recommended it to me four years ago because of the goodness in it, and I enjoy it, although I always like to eat something savoury with it, like nuts or crisps, which are usually in the house for nibbling anyway.

"By ten o'clock I'm beginning to get peckish again, so I might make myself some sandwiches or cheese on toast. Since I stopped work last year I can afford to go to bed at 10.30 or 11pm and still get my full 10 hours' sleep. Actually, I find that eating a snack that late helps me get over the weak feeling of hunger on my pre-breakfast run next morning.

"I do have a ritual pre-race meal of honey sandwiches with a cup of coffee, and I also take supplements of Vitamin C and multi-vitamins with iron. I may not need them now, but it started when I used to get in from training exhausted at 8pm, after a long day at work, and was too tired to cook a meal. It wasn't fair on the rest of the family to expect them to wait for me, so my meal always used to be re-heated, which meant that some of the goodness was lost, so the supplements were really to compensate.

"In total I run about 70 miles a week, and I'm fortunate that I've never had a weight problem. I've never been heavier than 7½ stone, and tend to vary between 7st and 7st 4lb now. But I often wonder what would happen if I stopped running and kept eating the same amount !"

Mike Gratton

Mike Gratton, 29, champion marathon runner, eats and drinks about 4,200 calories on an average day – more than men who do the heaviest kind of manual work, such as coal mining, forestry or farming. And it is almost twice the consumption of a man who has a sedentary job and does not exercise – yet Mike never puts on any weight. Mike eats quite a lot of empty calories in the form of sweet drinks and confectionery. With his high calorie requirement he is able to do so without seriously depriving himself of nutrients.

Mike won the 1983 London Marathon and was a bronze medallist in the 1982 Commonwealth Games. Formerly a schoolteacher, he now runs full time, supported by training grants, and lives in Canterbury.

"I wake up with my first cup of tea (with two sugars) around 8.30, then have the second with a bowl of cereal and sliced banana for breakfast before my morning training run, which might be five to 10 miles during the week, or 22 miles on a Sunday.

"At 11 o'clock I have a mid-morning cup of tea with four or five biscuits, and possibly a fruit yoghurt if I'm really hungry. Then I walk into town to buy the ingredients for the evening meal. I like to get fresh foods and cook them myself, but as I walk back from the shops I always eat a bar of chocolate, a Mars or Marathon, or Marks and Spencer's soft centred chocolate.

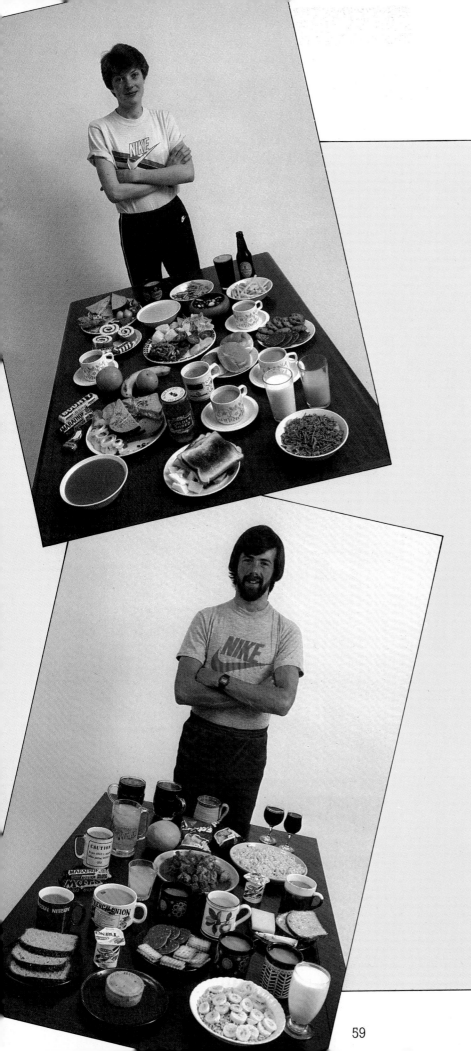

"You can't eat too much during the day because a very heavy meal would not digest properly before the next training session, so for lunch I have a large bowl of soup, with two or three slices of bread. I prefer brown bread, simply to follow normal dietary advice. I may have a pork pie too, followed by another fruit yoghurt, strawberry or banana flavoured.

"Mid-afternoon, around 3 o'clock, I'll have a couple of slices of toast or bread with a slab of Stilton. Even though cheese is a slow digesting food, I seem to be able to get away with training quite soon after eating it.

"The second training session is harder, faster and may involve repetitions, like 15 times 300 metres with a 100 metre jog on a track, or it could be another long run of 10 to 15 miles. When I've finished a long run I always drink a pint of orange squash straight away, and follow it up with tea and biscuits while I prepare the evening meal, which might be a large plateful of some vegetable curry of my own concoction, including carrots, onions, mushrooms, tomatoes, cauliflower, green peppers, pineapple chunks and raisins.

"I enjoy cooking, and it helps because my fiancée Debi, who lives in the same house, is busy at college all day. We usually wash down the meal with half a bottle of home-made red wine which Debi's father makes, with some fresh fruit for dessert. We don't eat many cakes, but perhaps twice a week we'll go down to the local pub afterwards, and there I'll usually drink two pints of bitter and eat several bags of crisps.

"By the end of the week, when the fatigue of training is catching up with me, I sometimes get a bit tired of preparing evening meals, and may succumb to the temptation of fast food. Then it's round to the fish and chip shop or McDonald's.

"Finally, I have a cup of coffee before bed around 11 pm, and, thinking about it, I get through a lot of liquid in a day, replacing the sweat lost from running 120 miles a week. But I don't worry about my weight. It's steady at around 10½ stone for my 5ft 10½ ins, though it may come down three or four pounds nearer to a marathon, when I'm training harder, and go up when I ease down training. But I don't really need scales to tell me when I'm heavier. I can tell just by the way I'm running."

Jane Furniss and Mike Gratton with the food they eat in one day.

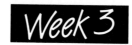
CONSUMPTION

The Constant Energy Diet

The basic principles of the Constant Energy Diet are as follows:
1 Cut out all 'overload foods' – sweet foods which cause hunger again within an hour or two, or rich foods loaded with high-calorie fat. You will have started to do this already over the last two weeks.
2 Balance your energy intake by eating some slow-release foods such as oats, rice, pasta or beans at each meal if you possibly can. You have already started to do this too.
3 Eat fat combined in small amounts with carbohydrate foods such as bread and potatoes – not too much and not too little, as we will explain.

1. Overload foods

Most overload foods are highly processed and so cause problems for the body. Highly refined carbohydrate foods cause a surge of glucose into the blood. As a result, too much insulin is produced and within an hour or two this is in turn causes the condition known as rebound hypoglycaemia – the removal of too much glucose from the blood. Hunger and tiredness may follow.

White bread, instant mashed potato, cornflakes and other heavily processed carbohydrate foods overload the body with refined starch. They are poorer in vitamins, minerals, fibre and protein and they usually cause a more rapid rise in blood glucose than the equivalent less refined, product. So you are asked to avoid them.

Other foods, such as sausages, pastries and biscuits, are included in the overload list because they provide the body with too much saturated animal fat, which is high in calories and bad for the heart, and sometimes too much sugar as well.

Fruit juices, like sweetened drinks, contain a lot of sugars in liquid form which pass through the stomach very quickly and are soon absorbed into the blood. This is why fruit juices are not advised in the Constant Energy Diet except

when well diluted or taken with other food. Instead, you should eat whole fruit, which release energy much more slowly than juices, because the cell walls of the fruit are broken down slowly in the body and sugars are leached into the blood in a steady flow. Apples are a particularly good slow-release fruit.

OVERLOAD FOODS

Cut these foods out of your diet or eat only in small quantities

beer
biscuits except when made with little sugar
bread, white
buns, sweet
cakes except when made with half normal sugar
cereals, breakfast, if sugared or not wholemeal
chocolates
cheese, cream
cocktail savoury snacks
cornflakes
cream
crisps
croissants
fruit juice except when well diluted with water
fruit tinned in syrup
honey – except in small quantities
ice cream
jam – except when made with reduced quantity of sugar or preserves made with no sugar
marmalade – except when made with reduced quantity of sugar
meats, processed
nuts, salted
pastry except for fruit pies etc.
pâtés
pies and tarts unless lightly sweetened
potato, instant mashed
puddings except when made with half normal sugar
Rice Crispies
salami
sausages
soft drinks
sweetened drinks
soups with added cream
sugar – except in small quantities
Sugar Puffs
sweets
syrup – except in small quantities
treacle – except in small quantities

2. Achieving energy balance

A healthy person who takes plenty of exercise can manage perfectly well by eating only fast release foods but may well have to eat between meals to avoid hunger and tiredness. There is nothing wrong with this so long as portions are moderate, but the danger is that large or even moderate meals plus snacks lead to excessive energy intake and in the long run to weight gain. This is especially likely when the snacks are of the sweet kind which overload the

system and lead to rebound hunger before the next meal.

Eating wholemeal rather than white bread is good for health and, because the fibre is filling and chewy, is helpful to slimmers. But eating wholemeal bread and foods with added fibre is not sufficient in itself to slow down energy release and prevent rebound hunger. Bread releases energy fast, while spaghetti and other pastas release energy relatively slowly, yet both are made from wheat. The reason for this is simple. Real pasta is made from semolina, which is a very coarsely ground flour and is not baked at high temperature like bread. More of the structure of the carbohydrate particles is preserved in pasta and it therefore takes longer to digest.

Cooking breaks down the cell walls of vegetables, making the sugars readily available. Raw carrots are a good slow-release food, whereas cooked carrots, especially if they are young, flood the body with sugar, if you eat enough of them, in just the same way as cornflakes or fruit juice.

FAST RELEASE FOODS

Try to combine in meals with slow release foods

bananas
beetroot
bread, wholemeal (or white)
carrots – unless raw
crispbreads eg Ryvita, waterbiscuits
muesli if sweetened
parsnips – unless raw
potatoes
Shredded Wheat
swedes – unless raw
Weetabix

3. Carbohydrate and fat in your diet

What is unique about the Constant Energy diet is that it gives guidance on combinations of food which postpone hunger, minimize fatigue and reduce any unnecess-ary calorie load. This is done by including some slow release carbohydrate in every meal and by combining fast release carbohydrates with a little fat.

Fats are high in calories and should therefore be eaten in small amounts only. But they slow down the speed at which food passes out of the stomach into the small intestine and therefore play an important part in preventing hunger. The key to feeling satisfied is to eat meals that contain at least one slow release food and some fat.

Avoid the extremes: Do not be tempted to eat, say, a large hunk of cheese or half an avocado pear at one sitting – always eat smaller amounts of fatty foods combined with carbohydrates. Eat less cheese with bread or a biscuit, or cook it in a sauce with vegetables – and prepare the avocado in a mixed salad.

Do not try to slim with the very low fat diets which advocate dishes such as cottage cheese and pineapple on unbuttered wholemeal toast. If you do, you are likely to suffer rebound hunger before long.

SLOW RELEASE FOODS

Try to include some of these in every meal

apples – raw	pasta white or
beans, dried, of all	wholemeal
kinds eg butter	peaches – raw
beans, haricot	pears – raw
or kidney beans	peas, frozen but
breads made with	not petit pois
wholegrains	peas, split
such as	porridge oats –
pumpernickel	cooked or
or German style	uncooked
heavy rye bread	rice – white or
(volkornbrod)	brown
lentils of all kinds	spaghetti – white
macaroni – white	or wholemeal
or wholemeal	sweetcorn
milk	yoghurt

WHAT ABOUT POTATOES?

Potatoes are a much misunderstood food. They are actually a good source of nutrients, a valuable source of good quality protein and fibre. And potatoes need not be any more fattening than many other foods. Potatoes should be eaten with *some* fat, because they are a fast release food and therefore increase the blood sugar rapidly; also, eating potatoes with some butter is much more appetising.

The Constant Energy Diet encourages you to combine baked jacket potatoes with butter or melted cheese to produce a satisfying and enjoyable meal. This should be done in a judicious way so that no more butter is used than is needed. Roast potatoes and even potato chips – provided they are cut very large – may be eaten within reason on the Constant Energy Diet, because the amount of fat (and the calories) absorbed by a potato increases as the potato is cut up smaller.

Potato crisps soak up fat like blotting paper: half a pound contains more than 1,200 calories, whereas a half pound baked potato contains only 170 calories and even with butter (level tablespoonful) still amounts to only about 300 calories. Average chips contain twice as many calories (about 80 per ounce) as thick cut chips, large cut roast potatoes, or sauté potatoes (about 40 calories per ounce). Crinkle cut chips or fine cut chips contain even more calories.

Cook your own large chips by cutting a medium sized potato lengthways into four, or make roast potatoes using large pieces. After cooking allow them to drain on kitchen paper before serving. When you mash potatoes add a little milk and a small knob of butter or margarine – it should make the meal more satisfying and help to postpone hunger.

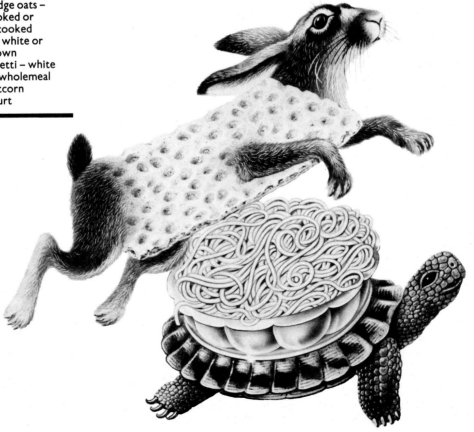

CONSUMPTION

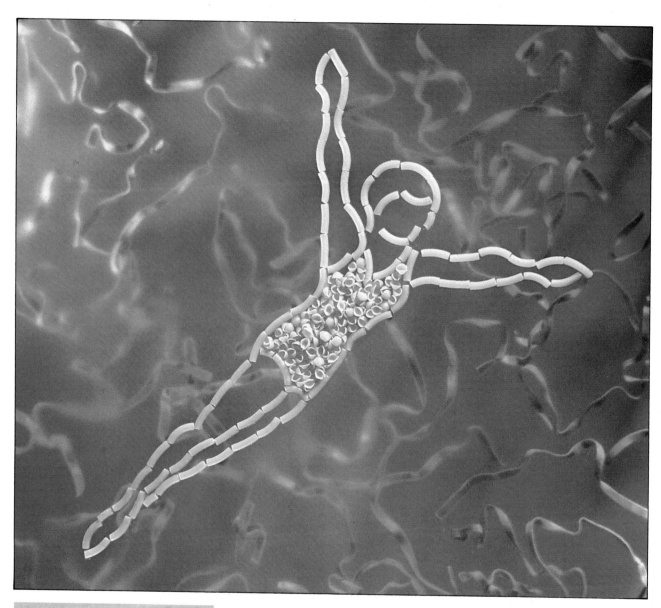

Pasta

In Britain and the United States pasta is thought of as being a fattening food, but many Italians defend it as good for those who want to lose weight. Generations of slimmers have mistakenly been told to cut pasta out of their diets because of its high carbohydrate content. However carbohydrate should form the basis of a healthy diet and, in fact, pasta is also a good source of protein. Weight for weight, pasta provides half as many calories as meat – so it is an excellent food for slimmers.

Pasta is digested slowly, which is helpful to hungry slimmers, and its high water content makes it filling. Ordinary Italian pasta does not contain bran but it does contain the wheat germ with its associated vitamins and so is not depleted in the same way as white bread. Southern Italians, who eat more pasta, vegetables and bread and less fat than Northern Italians, are less prone to heart disease. So pasta is high on the list of healthy foods.

Wholemeal pasta containing bran is now readily available, but with the bran comes extra phytate; so although you increase your fibre intake by eating wholemeal pasta you may also lose minerals, especially if you take extra bran in your diet, and this could make slimming more difficult.

Make sure you use Italian pasta, which is manufactured from semolina, a very coarse flour, according to strict controls, or choose a pasta which states on the packet that it is made from semolina including the wheat germ. Homemade pasta made from flour, although delicious, does not have the same slow energy releasing property. Although pasta will keep for two years or even longer it is best to use it as fresh as possible since the vitamin content drops and the flavour slowly deteriorates.

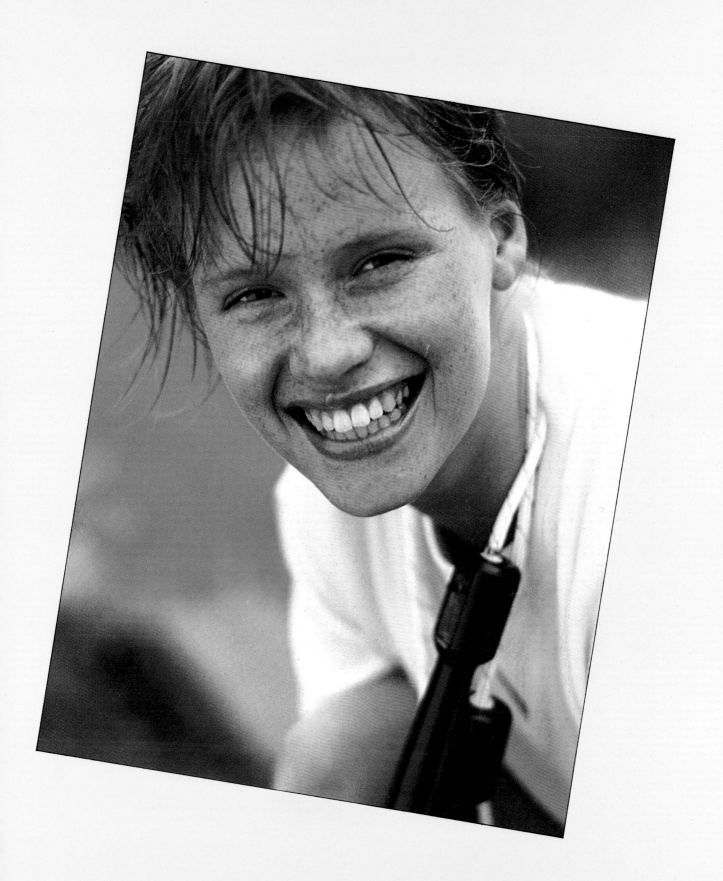

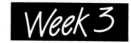

CONSUMPTION

Recipes

Tagliolini with Courgettes and Prawns

10oz (275g) fresh pasta (available at larger supermarkets) or 6oz (175g) dried pasta; 1lb (450g) small courgettes, cut into matchsticks or coarsely grated; 8oz (225g) frozen prawns; 2tbsp olive or sunflower oil; 1 clove garlic; salt and pepper; small knob of butter (optional). For the garnish: 2tbsp chopped dill; 1 lemon, quartered.

Heat the oil in a large heavy or non-stick pan and cook the crushed garlic briefly without browning it. Add the courgettes and cook them over a medium heat for a few minutes, tossing them with a wooden spoon so that they cook evenly. Put them in a serving dish in a warm oven, and heat the prawns gently in the juices that remain in the pan. Meanwhile, cook the pasta in plenty of boiling salted water. Mix together the prawns, courgettes and well drained pasta, season to taste and add a knob of butter if you like. Put back into the serving dish, sprinkle with chopped dill and put the lemon quarters round the dish.

Tagliolini is the fine, flat pasta. Ordinary spaghetti may be substituted but the dish won't be quite the same. For a special treat you could use smoked salmon. Cut the salmon into thin strips and warm gently in the oven with the cooked courgettes before mixing with the pasta.

Beef Casserole with Macaroni

This is a very filling Greek recipe which will happily cook while you are busy. Even at the end of the cooking time it can wait in a low oven for another half an hour if necessary.

1lb (450g) shin of beef or other lean stewing steak, cut into 1in (2.5cm) cubes; 12oz (350g) onions, sliced; 2 red peppers, seeded and chopped; 2oz (50g) back bacon or ham, cut into small pieces; 1 large orange, juice and grated rind; 2tbsp olive or sunflower oil; 1tbsp plain flour; 3/4 pint (400ml) stock, heated; 2 1/4 oz (60g) tin tomato purée; a glass of red wine, optional; bay leaf; salt and pepper; 12 olives; 6oz (175g) macaroni; 3 slices bread, grated into crumbs; a handful of parsley, chopped.

In a heavy casserole cook the onions and peppers in the oil until transparent but not brown. Remove from the pan with a slotted spoon and keep on one side. Cook the bacon in the same pan until just crisp, and set aside with the onion. Sprinkle the beef cubes with flour, and cook a few pieces at a time until brown on all sides. Return all the meat and vegetables to the casserole and add the tomato purée, dissolved in the hot stock, and the wine. Add the orange juice and half of the grated rind, the bay leaf and some pepper. Do not add any salt at this stage. Cover and cook in a low oven, 300°F (150°C, gas mark 2) for three hours.

While the casserole is in the oven cook the macaroni in plenty of boiling salted water, drain and put on one side. Combine the breadcrumbs, parsley and the rest of the grated orange peel. When the stew is tender remove from the oven, taste for seasoning, remembering that the olives you put in now will be salty. Ladle the stew into an ovenproof serving dish, alternating layers of stew and macaroni, ending with a layer of stew. Put the breadcrumb mixture over the top and put in a 350°F (180°C, gas mark 4) oven for 30-40 minutes. Serve with a green salad.

Tomato Sauce for Pasta

This sauce is good with all kinds of pasta and it combines particularly well with the cannelloni and gnocchi recipes

2lb (900g) ripe tomatoes, quartered or a large 1lb 14oz (850g) tin; 6oz (175g) onion, finely chopped; 4oz (100-125g) carrots, grated; 2tbsp olive or sunflower oil; 1 clove garlic; 2 1/4 oz (60g) tin tomato purée; salt and pepper; sugar (optional); fresh basil, marjoram or parsley, chopped.

Heat the oil in a heavy or non-stick pan. Cook the onion without browning until transparent, add the garlic and the carrot and cook a little longer. Add the tomatoes and the tomato purée and cook slowly for 30 minutes. Put the sauce into a food processor or rub through a sieve or Mouli-légumes; if it is too liquid reduce by cooking a little longer. Season with salt and pepper and a pinch of sugar if the sauce is too sharp. Add the fresh herbs at the end of the cooking time, but if you are forced to use dried ones add them 10 minutes or so before the sauce is cooked.

Cannelloni

16-18 cannelloni tubes or squares; 2lb (900g) fresh spinach or 1lb (450g) frozen spinach; 8oz (225) medium fat curd cheese plus 4oz (125g) fromage frais 0% fat or cottage cheese (or use 12oz (350g) ricotta cheese); 1 egg; 1/4tsp nutmeg; salt and pepper. For the top: 1oz (25g) Parmesan cheese, grated; tomato sauce (see recipe above)

Follow the instructions on the packet for the cooking of the cannelloni tubes or squares. If using the new instant type, do not prepare them too long in advance as they tend to disintegrate while standing. Wash, trim and drain the spinach, and cook it with just the water that clings to the leaves, adding a little salt. Cook frozen spinach following the instructions on the packet. When the spinach is tender, drain it in a sieve, pressing it hard to remove as much moisture as possible. Turn on to a board and chop the spinach finely. Combine the cheese, spinach, beaten egg and seasonings. Roll the filling up in the pasta squares or pipe it into the tubes. Place them in an oiled rectangular ovenproof dish or tin approximately 9in x 12in (22cm x 30cm). Pour the tomato sauce over the cannelloni and sprinkle with the grated Parmesan. Bake in the oven 350°F (180°C, gas mark 4) for 25-30 minutes.

Buckwheat Spaghetti with Spicy Sauce

This is a quick and easy meal. If you can get it, try to use fresh Parmesan grated from a lump rather than the small cartons. A piece of strong Cheddar which has become a little hard is a good substitute.

Tomato sauce (see recipe above); 4oz (100-125g) back bacon or lean ham, chopped; 2 red peppers; Tabasco or chilli sauce (optional); salt and pepper; 2oz (50g) Parmesan cheese, grated.

Fry the bacon or ham until crisp, and drain on kitchen paper. Grill the peppers until black and blistered and wrap them in a clean teatowel for 5 minutes. Remove the black skin, cut out the seeds, and chop the peppers. (If you have never done this before you will be surprised to find a subtle improvement in the flavour.)

Add the chopped peppers and bacon to the tomato sauce and cook for a few minutes to allow the flavours to mingle. Season the sauce and add a few drops of Tabasco or chilli sauce if you like the flavour.

The buckwheat spaghetti is very fine and needs only a few minutes' cooking in boiling salted water. Drain, transfer to a dish and stir in the sauce. Serve the Parmesan cheese separately.

Gnocchi

1 pint (600ml) milk; 7-8oz (200-225g) semolina; 1oz (25g) butter; 2 small eggs; 2oz (50g) Parmesan cheese, grated; 1/2 tsp grated nutmeg; salt and pepper; 1 bay leaf, broken into pieces.

Start to make this dish half a day before you want to eat it. Gently heat the milk with the bay leaf in a heavy saucepan. When the milk is hot remove the bay leaf, gradually whisk in most of the semolina, season with salt and pepper and slowly bring to the boil. Simmer the mixture for about 10 minutes, stirring all the time to avoid lumps. It should be about the same consistency as stiff mashed potato. If it is too runny add a spoonful or two more of the semolina, and cook a little longer. Remove from the heat, cool a few minutes then beat in the butter, eggs and half of the cheese. Spoon the mixture into an oiled Swiss roll tin 12in x 8in (25cm x 20cm) and spread out in an even layer, using a wet spatula. Allow to cool and refrigerate until needed.

Cut the gnocchi into 2in (5cm) squares and place them, slightly overlapping, in a fireproof dish. Sprinkle with the remaining cheese and bake in a moderate oven, 375°F (190°C, gas mark 5) for 25-30 minutes, until the top is crisp and golden. Alternatively the dish can be heated under a hot grill. The gnocchi can be served instead of potatoes as part of a larger meal or with tomato sauce (see recipe above) as a simple lunch or supper dish.

Spaghetti alla Carbonara

12oz (350g) packet spaghetti or 1lb (450g) fresh spaghetti; 6oz (175g) smoked back bacon (without rind) cut into 1/2in (1cm) squares; 2 tbsp olive oil; 1 clove garlic, crushed (optional); 4 eggs; 2oz (50g) Parmesan cheese, grated; 4 tbsp chopped fresh parsley; salt and freshly ground pepper.

Bring a large pan of salted water to the boil and cook the spaghetti cooked but firm to the bite (al dente). Meanwhile cook the bacon pieces in their own fat until crispy, then drain on kitchen paper. Heat the olive oil in the same pan and keep warm. Beat the eggs, half the cheese and parsley together with a pinch of salt and plenty of black pepper.

Drain the cooked spaghetti, quickly return it to the hot saucepan and stir in the egg mixture and the bacon, garlic and oil. Stir it all together for a moment so that the heat of the pasta and the pan cooks the eggs. Sprinkle with the rest of the cheese and serve on hot plates.

A sliced tomato salad with a little chopped onion makes this a good meal.

Rice with Omelette and Prawns

6oz (175g) rice, brown or white; 1 onion, finely sliced; 1 tbsp sunflower oil; 4oz (100-125g) french beans or frozen peas or sweetcorn; 4oz (100-125g) bean sprouts; 1in (2.5cm) piece of fresh ginger, grated (optional); 8oz (225g) frozen prawns; 2 tbsp soy sauce; 2 eggs; 4 spring onions.

Cook the rice with a little salt until just done. Meanwhile saute the onion in half the sunflower oil until brown, drain and keep hot. Toss the beansprouts and ginger in the rest of the hot oil until they are all hot and put these with the onions. Cook the peas, beans or sweetcorn until just done and put with the other vegetables. Heat the prawns briefly with the sherry: be careful they do not toughen through over cooking. Drain the rice when it is ready and mix in a large dish with the vegetables and the prawns, stir in the sesame oil and the soy sauce and keep hot. Quickly cook each beaten egg separately in a non-stick pan, making two thin flat omelettes. Shred these omelettes with a knife and chop up the spring onions. Arrange these on top of the dish and serve. A salad of shredded Chinese leaves with chopped green peppers and tomatoes would be nice with the dish.

Chicken Liver Risotto

The special rice for this dish is stocked by many delicatessens. If the chicken livers don't appeal to you, a little chopped ham, more mushrooms or fish may be used instead, or the rice with parmesan sprinkled over it could be served as part of a larger meal.

8oz (225g) Italian risotto (or arborio) rice; 12oz (350g) chicken livers, prepared and chopped; 1 onion, chopped; 2 cloves garlic, crushed; 4oz (100-125g) mushrooms, sliced; 4tbsp olive or sunflower oil; grated rind of 1 lemon; 1oz (25g) parmesan cheese, grated; about 2 pints (1.2 litres) stock; 2tbsp marsala or sherry; salt and pepper; 2-3 sage leaves, chopped.

Heat 2tbsp of the oil in a heavy or non-stick frying pan. Fry the onion until transparent and limp, add the garlic and mushrooms and cook for a moment or two longer before stirring in the rice. Continue to stir until the rice begins to look glossy. Measure the stock and heat it in another pan. (Use half a stock cube and a little tomato purée if you haven't any suitable stock). Add a ladleful or two of stock to the rice in the pan, and simmer gently until it is absorbed. Stir the rice occasionally and continue to add the hot stock, a little at a time, as it is absorbed by the rice. This will take approximately 20-25 minutes (the exact time will depend on the rice used).

Towards the end of the cooking time heat the rest of the oil in another pan and toss the chopped chicken livers until they brown. Add the marsala or sherry and the chopped sage leaves and let the pan bubble for a moment or two. When the rice is tender and most of the liquid has been absorbed, add the chicken livers and their juice, the lemon rind and the grated parmesan cheese and stir together (check the seasoning). Put the risotto into a warm serving dish and leave in a warm place for 3-4 minutes. Be careful not to overcook the chicken livers, or to cook them too long in advance as they will harden and become bitter.

YOUR ABC DIARY: Week Three					Starting date:			
	WALKING		JOGGING/ WALKING		SWIMMING		HOME WORKOUT	OTHER EXERCISE (e.g. cycling)
	Mins	Miles*	Mins	Miles*	Mins	Lengths	Mins	Mins
Monday								
Tuesday								
Wednesday								
Thursday								
Friday								
Saturday								
Sunday								
TOTAL								

* approximate distance, optional

ABC ROAD TEST	mins		mph				

BODY MEASUREMENTS	Date / /	Chest	Waist	Hips	Arms	Legs	Weight

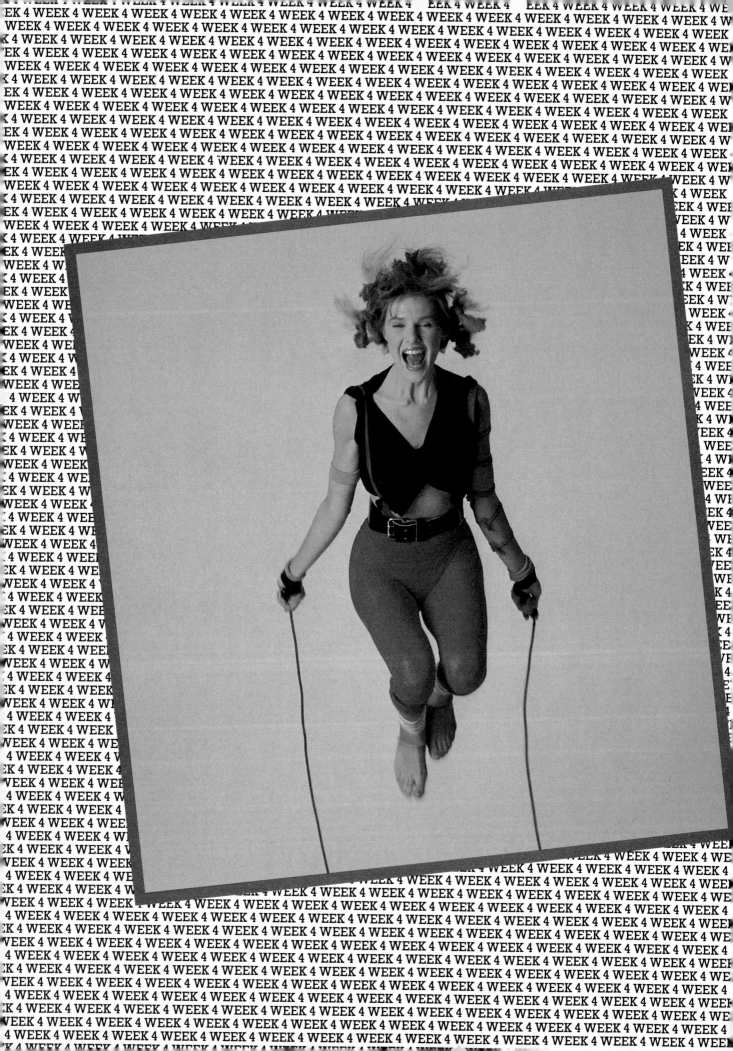

Week 4

A FOR ACTIVITY

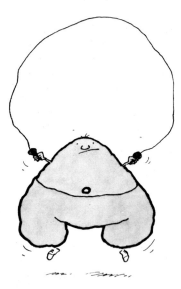

Choose five sessions of exercise this week, combining different types as you wish, but take care not to progress from one week to the next without doing at least three sessions of exercise at each level.

Do five exercise sessions this week.

Walking Programme

Walkers who started with a very slow walk of two miles an hour should be up to three or three and a half miles an hour by now, and may feel ready for a bit of limbering up. While out walking try jogging gently for 30 or 40 yards. If it feels good do a bit more but walk for two or three minutes to get your breath back between short runs.

You can gradually build up to jogging in this way, slowly increasing the amount you do. But avoid running up even small hills to begin with and stay within your capability. Gradually you will be able to spend more time jogging and less time walking. If you decide you want to jog, aim to pass the ABC Road Test then begin with Week One of Jogging 1.

There is no need to jog if you prefer walking. Walking is very good exercise and you should be able to reduce your body fat satisfactorily by walking if you persevere and combine it with the rest of the ABC Bodyplan. Fast walking at four or five mph uses up twice as much energy and burns twice as much fat as going at half the speed, so do not underestimate its value. Older people, and people who are infirm or very overweight, are advised to stick to walking or swimming; they are low-risk forms of exercise.

Jogging Programme

Jogging 1
- Walk briskly for about four minutes.
- Jog for two minutes, walk for two minutes. Do this six times, increasing to eight times during the week if you can. Take your pulse after the first three repeats to see if you are working hard enough (see Monitoring Progress, which follows below).
- Walk for up to 10 minutes, to give 40 minutes of exercise altogether. Finish off with the Cool Down Stretches.

Jogging 2
- Walk briskly for five minutes.
- Jog for five minutes, walk for five minutes. Do this three times. Take your pulse after the first repeat to see if you are working hard enough (see Monitoring Progress, which follows below).
- Walk for five minutes at the end.
- Finish with the Cool Down Stretches.

At the beginning of the week your jogs may be shorter – four or five minutes – but build to a seven minute jog by the end of the week if you can.

Swimming Programme

With swimming you have to build up your technique as well as your fitness, so progress may be a bit slow at first, but you can speed up by swimming harder now that your muscles are more accustomed to the new demands being made on them. Use your breathing and pulse as a guide, as for any other exercise (see Monitoring Progress, which follows below). Take your pulse after swimming three consecutive lengths and see if you should aim to be swimming at a faster pace.

Swimming 1
Warm-up
- Begin by swimming a few widths, trying to improve your strokes, or do the Pool Exercises. You can also try the Figure Trimming Exercises this week (see below), but leave the last two exercises to the more advanced swimmers for the time being.

Exercise
- This week aim to swim 14 lengths, alternating your preferred stroke with sidestroke or backstroke. Use the lengths of sidestroke and backstroke to work hard and get your pulse going fast. Stop to rest when you need to but try to increase the length of continuous swimming.
- End with the Pool Exercises.

Swimming 2
Warm up
- Swim two lengths of your first stroke just to warm up. Rest if you need to. Now practise two

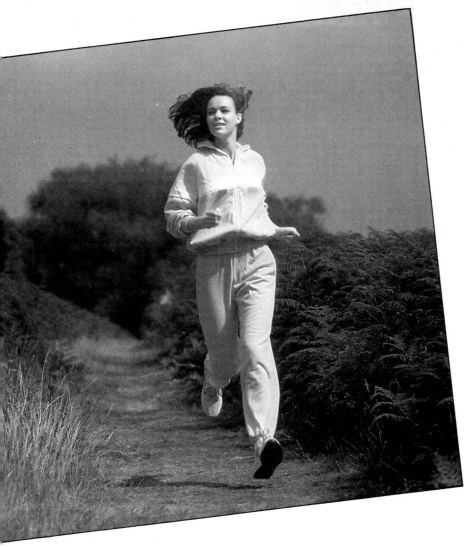

Stair climbing

If you have reached 200 steps in under two and half minutes, that is very good going. Maintain this steady speed and if you want to increase the demands made by this exercise, do it for longer – say three minutes or 300 steps.

Cool Down Stretches

Don't forget them.

Monitoring Your Progress

By observing your breathing or your pulse you can tell if your exercise is hard enough to burn fat.

Breathing

If you are breathing deeply after a few minutes' exercise, you have been exercising effectively. During exercise the body needs more oxygen because it is burning up more fuel to supply energy. Deep breathing does not mean gasping or panting – although you may well do a bit of that – but rather taking deep, rhythmic breaths. After brisk walking for five minutes or climbing stairs for one or two minutes you should be breathing deeply (but still able to talk or sing).

Pulse

As you exercise, your heart beats faster and is able to pump additional oxygenated blood from the lungs to the muscles, where the oxygen is needed to release energy. As your heart takes some time to slow down after you have been exercising, measuring your pulse immediately after gives a good indication of the intensity of the exercise. For there to be a training effect, it has been found that the pulse rate should be sustained for several minutes at between 70 and 90 per cent of the maximum. But unless you are very fit and under 30 you should not attempt to exercise at over 80 per cent of maximum. The maximum pulse rate varies with age as shown in the table, which also gives pulse rates to aim for in training.

lengths of your second stroke, concentrating on breathing and style.

Exercise

You have already swum four lengths; now swim another 18 lengths, alternating your first and second strokes with each other or with sidestroke or backstroke.
Stop and rest every four lengths or so if you need to.

The Home Workout

After two weeks of this plan you will be much fitter, so you can probably step up the plan from half an hour to 40 minutes four or five times a week without being too exhausted. Check your pulse from time to time (see Monitoring Progress) to know whether you are working hard enough. Divide the time as you wish between the different exercises but keep up a good pace and don't rest for long between exercises. Spend a few minutes on the Warm Up Exercises (Week Two) before you begin.

Dancing or room running

Try to develop a dancing or running pace which is demanding but which you can sustain for 10 minutes at a time. Extend the time you spend dancing to two 10 minute sessions. Do some room running as well, if you like. It is sustained exercise which is most effective.

Skipping

You have to twirl the skipping rope at least 80 times per minute to keep it from getting tangled up. This is equivalent to running a mile in seven minutes and 20 seconds – a creditable speed for an amateur athlete. Do not expect to be able to skip for very long periods of time; if you can manage a minute or two at a time you are doing well. You should have mastered the skipping two-step by now. Try doing it for about a minute (80 to 100 turns), stop for a short rest and continue for another minute. Then work on doing it for two minutes at a time. If the rope snags, just carry on as quickly as you can until the time comes for a break.

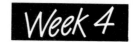

ACTIVITY

Take your pulse at the wrist or neck for 10 seconds after 10 minutes or so of your routine exercise, without resting first. Count it for 10 seconds and multiply by six. If it is below the 70 per cent of maximum recommended for training, see if you can get it up higher in the next 10 minutes of exercise by performing at a faster rate.

If you find that your pulse is above the 80 per cent maximum level, do not worry. Ease up a bit, because you have been trying too hard.

Five minutes after finishing your exercise your pulse should be below 120 beats per minute; 10 minutes after exercise it should be below 100. If your pulse does not go down in this way after exercise you should ease up and build your fitness more gradually.

Pulse (beats/minute) should be between 70 per cent and 80 per cent of maximum in order to have a training effect.

Age	Maximum pulse	Training range 70% of maximum	80 % of maximum
15	210	147	168
20	200	140	160
25	195	136	156
30	190	133	152
35	185	129	148
40	180	126	144
45	173	121	138
50	166	116	133
55	160	112	130
60	155	108	124
65	150	105	120

Maximum heart rates are slower during swimming, probably because heart function is altered by the position of the body. So swimmers should subtract 10 beats per minute from the minimum and maximum training pulse rates.

The pulse is only one guide to the effectiveness of training and you should not use it to push yourself harder if you are not feeling well or if you are suffering from any kind of injury to muscles or tendons. Exercise plans must be flexible and be adapted to how you feel.

How to Avoid Injury

Overdoing it

If you are doing too much all at once, you may become susceptible to injuries and minor illnesses. Fatigue, frequent colds, diarrhoea are warning signs. If you are caught up in other pressures you may have to ease up on your exercise schedule temporarily. Decrease the amount of running and do more walking, swim shorter distances, or make your Home Workout leisurely. If you feel really ill, stop altogether until you have recovered and start slowly again with relatively gentle exercises. If you find you have increased your level of exercise too quickly, fall back to a level you can manage.

Illness

If you have had an illness which keeps you in bed for two or three days, you should begin your exercise programme again in very easy stages. Joggers should begin again with walking.

If you are unsure whether you are just tired from stress at work or if you are unwell, go for a trial jog, swim or workout. After 10 minutes you may feel the stress lift and by the end of half an hour you will feel much better. But if after five or 10 minutes you are feeling much worse then stop, go home and get an early night. Rest the next day and try again after that if you are no worse.

Stretch out for flexibility

Remember to do the Cool Down Stretches given in Week One after your exercise session. This is essential to develop flexibility of the Achilles tendon, hip, back, calf and hamstring muscles.

What to Do About Injuries

This section tells you how to deal with the most common injuries suffered by joggers. It should not be used as a substitute for proper medical advice, however.

When you are injured

You must allow time for healing. A minor injury may become major if you neglect it. Recovery may be slow, so be prepared to take up walking, swimming or slow jogging to keep up the exercise while healing proceeds. Avoid running over hills and on hard ground – choose grass rather than roads – while recovering, and avoid running at speed and doing long distances.

Pain

Injuries should always be treated with ice first, as this contracts the blood vessels and prevents bleeding in the muscle. If it is a joint which has been injured, apply ice followed by compression with an elastic bandage. Finally, rest the injured limb in a raised position. If pain continues, see a physiotherapist recommended by your doctor.

Feet

Painful arches are a common problem. Help can be obtained by using running shoes which include an arch support, as most generally do. If the arch support in your running shoe does not seem adequate, you could try using a Dr. Scholl arch support, obtainable from chemists. If the feet are very painful you may have to rest temporarily. Do these strengthening exercises to improve and maintain arches.

Exercises

Pick up marbles with your toes, or stand on the edge of a book and press your toes down so that your arch lifts.

Heels

The Achilles tendon attaches the strong muscles of the lower leg to the heel. Injuries are painful and slow to heal. If the tendon is inflamed, it becomes painful and stiff after exercise and tender to the touch. Stop running for a couple of days at least – and for a week if necessary.

If the pain persists after a week then it is probably advisable to seek a medical opinion. Cortisone injections may bring dramatic relief but they are controversial and may make a rupture of the tendon more likely.

Slow down your programme at the first sign of strain in your Achilles tendon, but if it is not so bad as to prevent running

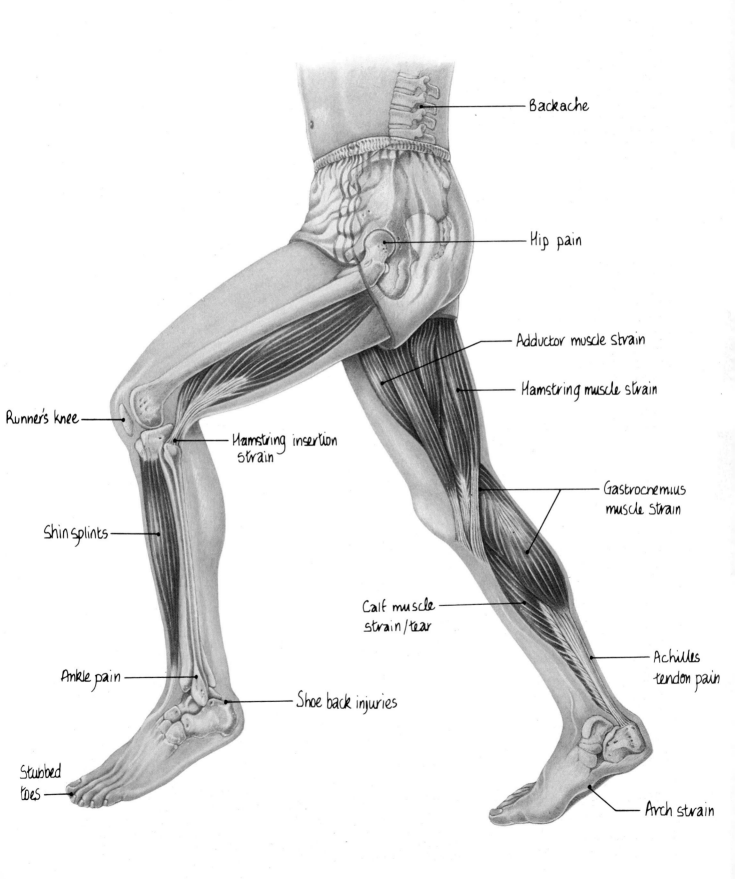

Backache

Hip pain

Adductor muscle strain

Hamstring muscle strain

Runner's knee

Hamstring insertion strain

Gastrocnemius muscle strain

Shin splints

Calf muscle strain/tear

Achilles tendon pain

Ankle pain

Shoe back injuries

Stubbed toes

Arch strain

ACTIVITY

altogether, treat the tender area with heat before exercise and with cold afterwards.

It will probably help to put some heel lifts in your running shoes as a temporary measure to take some of the strain off the tendon. Do not do any stretching exercises at this stage because it is probably excessive sudden stretching which has caused the problem in the first place. Keep up gentle exercise, if you can, by running on flat grass and only begin cautious stretching exercises after three or four weeks without pain.

Exercises
Do the Calf Stretch – see the Cool Down Stretches in Week One – at least twice a day as the injury heals.

Ankles

Ankle strain may affect those who are overweight or used to wearing high-heeled shoes. Sometimes the ankle becomes swollen as well as inflamed and painful. The same can happen to experienced runners when they trip or catch their foot in a pothole. First treat the ankle as described above under Pain. Stop running until it begins to improve, then go back and build up in easy stages. Swimming is useful at this stage because the ankle will be more comfortable when it is not carrying your weight.

If you have ankle problems then be sure to do these ankle exercises before running. Good shoes and special exercises will also help.

Exercises
Any exercises which stretch the Achilles tendon and calf muscles are likely to help with ankle problems – see exercises for shin splints and Achilles tendon problems. Mobilize the ankle by turning it in slow circles. This helps to strengthen it and give it flexibility. Knee and calf releases (Warm Up Exercises – Week Two) are also good for the ankle – do them regularly when ankles have recovered.

Shin Splints

This condition, common in novice runners, is a painful swelling of the muscles and tendons of the shin. If you suffer from shin splints there

may be an easy remedy:

- Running on your toes or the balls of your feet is a common reason for shin splints. Heel lifts in your shoes may help if you find it difficult to put your foot flat on the ground when running. Use them until stretching exercises make them unnecessary.
- Leaning forward while running is another possible cause. Do not hunch over; try to keep an upright posture.
- You may have tight calf muscles or short Achilles tendons – perhaps as a result of wearing high heels. This throws a strain on the front of the leg, but the problem can be remedied by stretching exercises for the Achilles tendon – see Heels above.
- Tight clothing round the waist or upper leg may restrict circulation and cause painful symptoms similar to shin splints.
- If you have weak arches your foot may be unstable when it hits the ground, leading to shin splints. Arch supports may help.
- Some people seem to curl their toes when the foot strikes the ground. Supports under the toes called 'anterior crests' may help prevent this problem - these may be made from chiropody felt, 'moleskin', or adhesive foam, available from chemists.

If you get severe shin splints rest for a couple of days and see a doctor if they do not get better. Meanwhile, try the following suggestions to bring relief:

- Rest on a settee with your feet up whenever you can.
- Massage the painful area with ice (or frozen vegetables) in a plastic bag.
- Put heel lifts or arch supports in your shoes temporarily. Manufactured by Dr. Scholl, these are available from chemists.
- Run on level grass until the problem resolves.

Exercises
To prevent shin splints it is important to stretch the hamstrings and the calf muscles. Make sure you do Cool Down Stretch 3.

Pulled muscles

Stiffness is very common among

beginners. When legs have not been exercised for years they have to adapt to the new stresses put on them. Some stiffness is normal when training but if it seems excessive, then do not increase your times or distances until it begins to ease. Hot baths are an excellent way of relieving sore muscles, and long warm-ups and stretching before running also help, especially in cold weather. Spend more time on warm-ups when it is cold.

If a muscle is actually pulled, ice in a plastic bag applied to it will help to relieve the pain. Rest with the leg up as often as you can for 48 hours following the pull. Gentle massage may help. Return to light exercise – walking and possibly swimming – before running again.

Knees

Knee injuries are common among joggers. One cause is what running experts call over-pronation – a tendency to put too much weight on the inside of the foot.

You can tell if you do this by studying your shoes. If there is more wear on the inside than on the outside then you are an over-pronator. Arch supports such as Dr Scholl's may help to stabilize the leg at the knee and prevent over-pronation. Also continue doing the arch exercise described in the section on Feet above.

Seek out a soft even surface for running if you are having knee problems. An elasticated knee support may also be helpful.

Running in such a position that the legs are never fully extended – perhaps because of tight hamstrings – can be another cause of knee injuries.

Exercises
Inflexibility of the knee and tight leg muscles are potential causes of knee problems. These flexibility and strengthening exercises for the knee can help.

- To strengthen the muscles which support the knees (quadriceps), sit on a table or chair. Lift one leg at a time, keeping the foot flexed, toes pulling up towards you. As strength increases add some weight to the end of the leg such as heavy shoes.

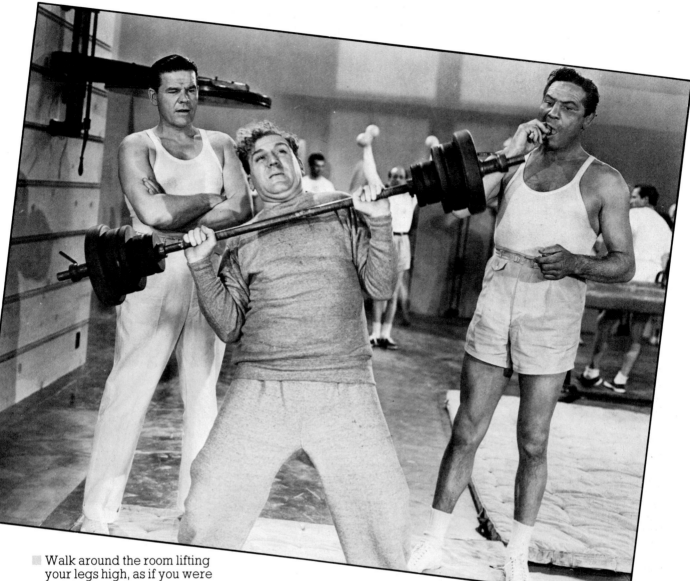

Max Baer in 'The McGuerins From Brooklyn'.
(United Artists, 1942)

- Walk around the room lifting your legs high, as if you were walking in water.
- Walk up and down the stairs whenever you get the opportunity.
- To stretch the quadriceps, do Cool Down Stretch 5 twice daily.
- To stretch the hamstrings do Cool Down Stretch 3 twice daily.

Hips

Hip pain is often the result of another problem such as weak feet, poor shoes or unequal leg length. See discussion of these problems under Back and Feet. Running on slanted or uneven surfaces can make it worse, so always work out on good surfaces. Stretching and strengthening hip muscles will help.

Exercises

- Stand sideways to a wall with one arm stretched out towards it and lean against the wall. Press the hip closest to the wall in towards the wall and hold for 25 seconds. Repeat several times with each side.
- To strengthen the hips, lie on your left side on the floor, using your top arm for support and your bottom arm to prop up your head. Make sure your top hip is directly above the bottom hip. Lying on a soft surface such as a carpet makes this more comfortable. Bend your left leg to help stabilize the position. Lift the top leg up with the knee facing forward. Lift the leg up so that you feel the muscles in the outside thigh and around the hip joint contract. Do this 10 times at first and build up. Bend top leg to release muscles and repeat on the other side. This will also help tighten buttocks.

Back

Bad backs are a very common problem among people who start any exercise programme because the postural muscles which keep the back in position have become weakened through neglect. Being overweight exacerbates the problem. If the stomach sticks out, it distorts balance by making it necessary to lean slightly backwards, which puts a strain on the back.

Some stiffness and aching in the back is normal when you start to exercise and after long runs. But if it is severe, you should rest for a few days and take hot baths to relieve it. Gradually return to running but spend less time running and more time walking to begin with. At the same time take up muscle strengthening and relaxation exercises.

A C T I V I T Y

Weak abdominal muscles and lack of flexibility are a common cause of back problems in people who have not been accustomed to taking exercise. Exercises for the abdominals are especially beneficial for people who are fat and have a protruding belly.

How to test for possible causes of back pain:

1. Weak abdominal muscles

If you cannot get off the floor in the bent knee curl-up exercise (The Home Workout – Week Seven) without your tummy quivering or feeling a pull in your lower back, your abdominal muscles are weak. During running these muscles will not support your body properly and as a result your pelvis will tilt forward, causing a sway back.

2. Lack of flexibility

Running actually decreases flexibility because it tightens calf and hamstring muscles. Flexibility can prevent and relieve back pain, so it is a good plan to do regular stretching exercises before and after running. If you are not able to rest your leg on a very low surface without feeling a strong pull up the back of your thigh during Cool Down Stretch 3 the hamstring muscles are too tight. Do this stretch twice daily.

3. Unequal leg length

Test for this by sitting on the floor with your legs straight out in front and your lower back flat against a wall. The ankle bones should come together if the legs are the same length. Many people with one leg slightly longer than the other have

no trouble and should do nothing. However, it is possible that this asymmetry is putting a strain on your back when you run. Try inserting a sole or heel lift in the shoe of the shorter leg. If this improves matters, leave it in. (A bad back may, of course, get better spontaneously, so you can't be certain that this is the answer unless the trouble begins to return when you try taking it out.)

Weak feet, poor shoes, leaning forward too much when running, and incorrect lifting techniques are all causes of back pain. When lifting, be certain to keep your back straight, stay close to the object to be lifted and bend your knees so that you are using the power of your legs rather than your back. Get a hard mattress or

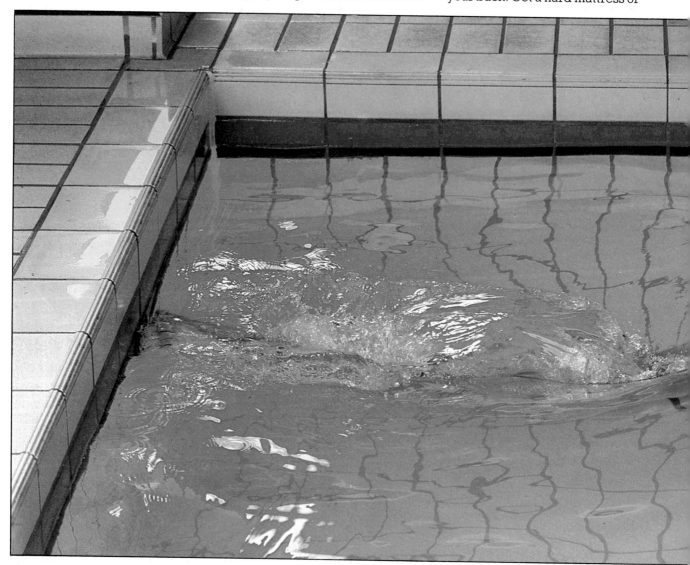

put a board under your present mattress. If back pain is a persistent problem seek medical advice and get in touch with the Back Pain Association (Grundy House, 31-33 Park Road, Teddington, Middlesex TW11 OAB), who can provide a wealth of practical advice.

Exercises

1) For the abdominals

- Stand in a comfortable position. Tighten all your abdominal muscles, pulling in the tummy as you breathe out; hold for about five seconds. Release as you breathe in. Repeat about 10 times.
- Lie on the ground with your legs together and slightly bent, your arms at your sides. Pull in your tummy muscles so that you feel your lower back press down into the floor. Raise your head and upper back from the ground and hold for a few seconds, whilst breathing out. Release while breathing in, and repeat. Eventually you will be able to sit up fully with your arms at your side. Continue with this exercise until you can do it at least five times, then start doing it with your arms folded across your chest. When you can do five folded-arm curl-ups, you can attempt the full curl-ups with arms behind the head, as described in the Home Workout in Week Seven.

2) For flexibility in the lower back

- Try the 'cat back' exercise. Get down on your hands and knees. Pull in your tummy, tucking your chin in so that your back rounds up, and breathe out. Release as you breathe in, allowing your back to hollow and lifting your head.
- Stand with feet slightly apart, hands on hips. Lift the right hip and heel, feeling the waist muscles 'pull up' on the right and release on the left. Lower the right hip and heel and raise the left hip and heel. Repeat slowly several times, then faster. Do not move the top half of your body.

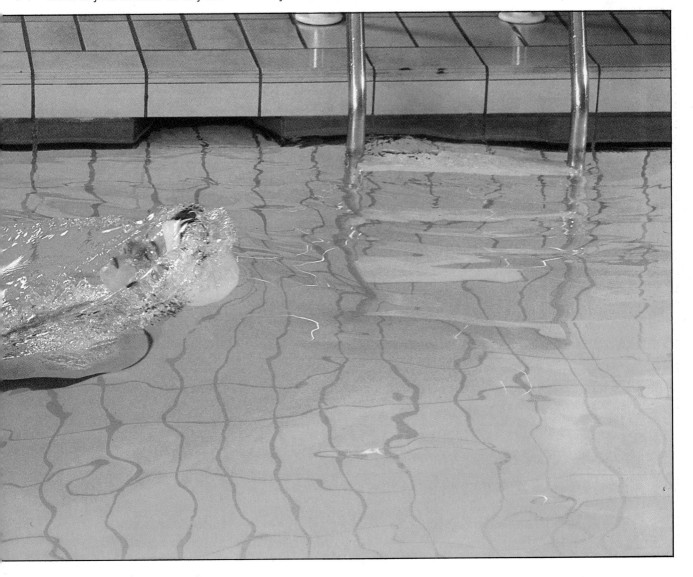

B FOR BEHAVIOUR

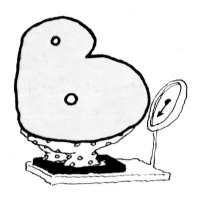

Tension Control

You have a choice of two very effective techniques to pick from – a sequence of tense-and-release exercises or simple meditation. The exercises work directly on the main muscle groups, on the principle that anxiety and muscular tension are inseparable. The meditation relieves stress by reducing the level of background 'noise' in the nervous system. This 'noise' is present all the time, but too much of it can hinder the smooth functioning of the nervous system, just as interference to radio waves hinders clear transmission.

Deep relaxation, a skill which needs to be learned and practised, will enhance your sense of control in several ways:
- *by curbing bad habits* such as overeating, drinking too much or smoking. 'Tension control reduces harmful displacement activities resulting from nervousness, particularly excessive eating and anxiety nibbling,' says Dr Malcolm Carruthers, a pathologist at the Maudsley Hospital in London and a leading figure in the field of stress management.
- *by making you more aware of your body's needs,* including the difference between false and true appetite.
- *by giving the body a chance to regulate itself.* Tension release switches off the body's alarm, the sympathetic nervous system, which prepares us for fight or flight, and allows the opposing system, the parasympathetic, to take over. The latter is responsible for the peaceful activities of rest, digestion and healing.
- *by making you feel more energetic and confident.* 'Your energy reserves and vitality are raised when you control stress, so that your body image improves and confidence is boosted,' according to Dr. Carruthers.
- *by making you better able to tolerate all forms of stress,* whether physical (eg viruses, sudden temperature changes, overwork) or psychological (eg hostility, discomfort, disappointment). Regular deep relaxation acts as stress-proofing.

Overeating, heavy drinking and smoking are some of the most common ways in which we attempt to cope with tension; they are damaging to health both because of the direct physical effects they have and because they are habits that reduce our sense of control over our lives.

This sense of being in control, of feeling that we are acting out of choice and can influence events, is beginning to emerge as the single most important prerequisite for mental and physical well-being. A number of studies by doctors and psychologists around the world have shown that a perception of helplessness may play a part in causing illness and can influence the eventual outcome. Cancer, diabetes, severe depression and stress are all cases in point. A sense of powerlessness may also be the critical factor in preventing people from slimming successfully.

You have already made a major move towards taking control of your weight and well-being by embarking on the ABC Diet and Bodyplan. This week introduces tension control as another step towards gaining control over your life.

● *by making you less likely to over-react emotionally.* Relaxation lowers the physiological arousal that triggers emotions. So you will feel calmer and more efficient.

● *by establishing a hotline to the unconscious.* When we are deeply relaxed, we are also more suggestible than in normal consciousness. Relaxation can be used as a first step in reprogramming the human computer. Later in the book we show you how to do this by giving yourself positive suggestions, and by using imagery to visualize the way you want to be.

Which method should you go for?

If you have high blood pressure, avoid the tense-and-release exercises and instead practise meditation, an effective way of reducing high blood pressure. If you already use a relaxation or meditation technique which is different from the ones outlined in this book, carry on using it unless you particularly want to change. Otherwise choose whichever method you prefer.

Tense-and-Release Exercises

These are best done lying down in a warm, quiet room with dimmed lights. But they can also be done sitting down.

Lying down: Lie on the floor, preferably on a rug or blanket, arms by your side but not touching the body, feet pointing outwards. If your neck needs support, use a cushion or pillow or, better still, a book or books about 2½ inches thick. If you have a sway back or pain in your lower back, put a pillow under your knees to take the strain off the lumbar region, and keep them slightly bent.

Sitting: Sit with your lower back supported. If the chair has no headrest to lean back against, you will need to clasp your hands behind your neck in order to tense your neck muscles.

How to do them: Work from top to toe, tensing and releasing each muscle group in turn. Hold each position for about 10 seconds, then release. Pay attention to the muscles relaxing and make a mental note of what it feels like for specific muscle groups to let go. After about 15 seconds, move on to the next group.

1. Eyes and forehead. Close eyes, screw them up tight, frown hard.

2. Jaw and tongue. Clench jaw, press tongue against roof of mouth.

3. Neck. Press head against floor, pillow or seat, or clasp hands behind head and press head against hands.

4. Shoulders back. Draw shoulders back, as though trying to make shoulder blades touch.

5. Shoulders up. Hunch shoulders, as though trying to touch ears.

6. Arms. Straighten arms, clench fists, tighten arm muscles.

7. Abdomen. Draw in abdominal muscles, as though trying to touch spine with abdomen.

8. Buttocks. Squeeze buttocks together.

9. Legs. Straighten legs, bend back feet, tighten leg muscles.

10. Toes. Scrunch up toes and squeeze.

11. Checking. Check that eyes, forehead, jaw and tongue are relaxed without tensing these muscles first.

12. Verbal suggestion. Say to yourself: 'I am completely relaxed from my head to my knees to my toes' as you feel a wave of warmth and relaxation wash over you from head to foot.

Afterwards: At the end of the sequence you should be feeling warm and very comfortable, as well as refreshed; you may even have a sensation of almost floating.

When to do them: Do these exercises at least once a day, preferably twice, any time you feel under pressure, anxious, aching or tired. After a hard day they can be as restorative as a nap.

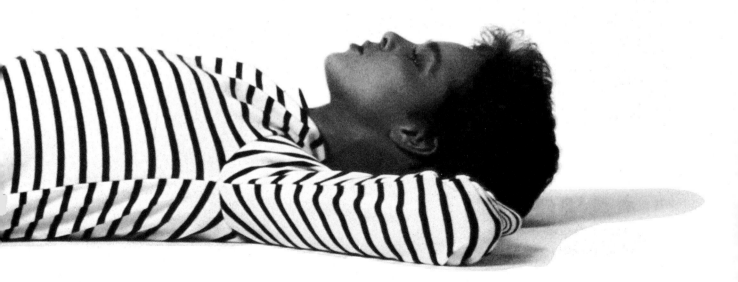

BEHAVIOUR

Simple Meditation

This technique, an alternative to the tense-and-release exercises, should be practised in a sitting position. The spine should be straight and the lower back supported. Low lighting and minimal distractions are a help: take the telephone off the hook.

The essence of meditation is an attitude of passivity. Sit quietly, hands resting loosely on your lap, close your eyes and simply observe your breathing. Do not attempt to make it slower or faster, deeper or shallower. Just pay attention to the rhythm as you inhale and exhale.

At the end of the relaxation, before getting up, repeat the following words to yourself: 'I am completely relaxed from my head to my knees to my toes' and at the same time feel a sensation of warmth and relaxation. Repeat twice. Wait a few moments before opening your eyes.

During the meditation, keep movements to a minimum but do not strain to stay still. If you must, for example, scratch you nose, do so unhurriedly and return to meditating. When thoughts intrude, don't try to drive them out: any wilful effort straight away creates tension. As to 'making your mind blank', which is what many tracts on meditation advise, don't even bother because if you've ever tried you'll know it's an impossibility, a contradiction in terms. Instead simply bring your attention back to your breathing. You may feel happy or sad, bored or angry, but you should not judge what is happening or try to inhibit feelings: simply accept them and return to your breathing.

The experience of meditation is different for everyone. You can expect to feel calmer, more clear-headed and generally better disposed towards the world. But the physical effects of de-stressing in this way vary. You may find yourself able to sit up with a straight back more easily or you may get rumblings in your tummy as tension in your gut is released. You may become aware of tension you didn't know you had in your neck and shoulders and feel like following up the meditation with some gentle stretching.

Practise at least once a day, preferably twice, for at least 10 minutes each time but no more than 20. Wait at least half an hour after eating. A good time to do it is before meals.

Shortcut to deep relaxation

Whichever method of tension control you use, after a few days you will be familiar with the sensation of deep relaxation. You will then be able to produce the sensation at will by simply closing your eyes, repeating the phrase 'I am completely relaxed from my head to my knees to my toes' as you relax. This is a useful shortcut when you haven't the time for a complete session and can be used at any time of the day.

Eliminating Tension at Source

If you lead a very stressful life, you will certainly benefit from practising one of the relaxation techniques and from regular exercise. But you should also try to eliminate some of the stress at source.

- Allow yourself some time alone every day, even if it's only 15 minutes, and take a short break every hour or so.
- Establish your priorities. Writing them down will help.
- Do just one thing at a time. Shaving while you're cooking the toast and trying to catch the 8 o'clock news may save some time, but it's a false economy.
- If you are feeling swamped by the magnitude of a task, be analytical: break it down into manageable proportions.
- Learn to delegate and to ask for help (don't always ask the same person).
- Be prepared to lower your standards if necessary: doing an adequate job is much less stressful than trying to be perfect, and it may be more important to get the job finished.
- If you're often asked to do favours you would rather not do, learn to say no without feeling guilty.
- Learn to recognize your emotions and to find appropriate ways of expressing them instead of bottling them up because you feel they're unacceptable.

Additional help

Tapes: 'Just Relax', a guided meditation by healer Matthew Manning, for morning and evening use. £3.95 from 39 Abbeygate Road, Bury St. Edmunds, Suffolk IP33 1LW. 'Relax and Enjoy It', a sequence of clench-and-release exercises by psychologist Dr. Robert Sharpe. £6.00 from Lifeskills, 3 Brighton Road, London N2 8JU.

Courses: Details of relaxation courses from local library or Relaxation for Living, 29 Burwood Park Road, Walton-on-Thames, Surrey. Details of meditation courses from Siddha Yoga Dham, 15 Fitzroy Square, London W1P 5HQ or Transcendental Meditation National Office, Roydon Hall, East Peckham, Tonbridge, Kent (for London courses, contact centres listed in directory under Transcendental Meditation).

Books: Stress and Relaxation by Jane Madders (Martin Dunitz), Simple Relaxation by Laura Mitchell (John Murray).

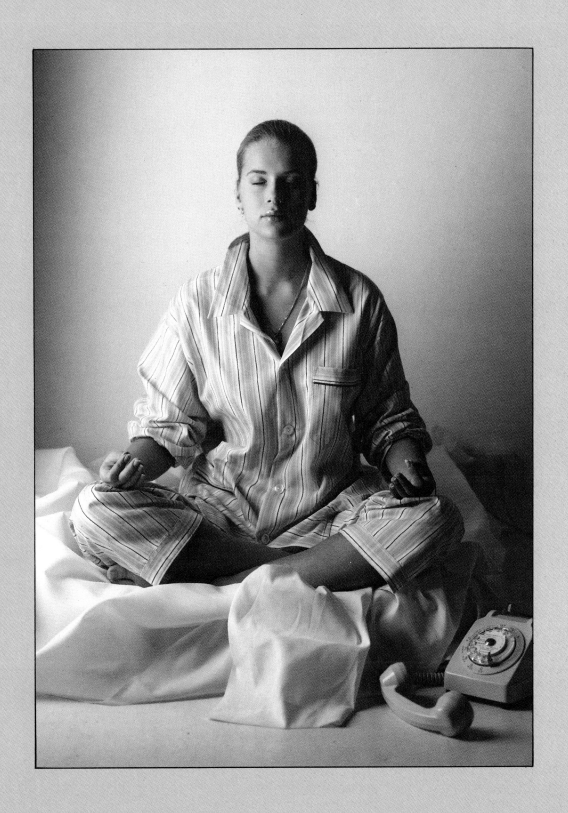

C FOR CONSUMPTION

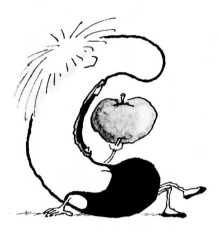

An individual only needs one tablespoon of fat or oil per day in order to remain healthy. This small amount is necessary because the human body cannot make all the different constituents, including certain vitamins, which are obtained from fat or oil. However, most people eat six or seven times as much fat (or oil) as they need. Some of this is used up as energy; the surplus is stored as body fat.

ALL CALORIES ARE NOT EQUAL

A fatty diet is more likely to make a person fat. Fat in the diet can be taken up directly by the body's fat stores, whereas carbohydrate has to be converted into fat. This means that for 100 calories of carbohydrate about a quarter is lost as energy in the conversion. So if you switch from a diet with a high proportion of fat to one with a high proportion of carbohydrate you can, for this reason alone, eat the same number of calories and lose weight. Furthermore people eating a diet containing a high proportion of carbohydrate burn up more energy during their sleep.

Fat Puts on Inches

Most people do not realize how much fat they eat because it is hidden in foods that are generally regarded as nourishing. Meat, for example, generally contains more fat than protein: 100 grams of beef sirloin contains 23 grams of fat and 17 grams of protein, and even if all the visible fat is cut off, in terms of calories the remaining meat will still be 42 per cent fat. Cheaper cuts of meat have an even higher fat content – mince, for example, contains almost equal amounts of protein and fat by weight and, in terms of calories, is 65 per cent fat.

Cheese, though often thought of as a protein food, is also high in fat. Cheddar contains 34 grams of fat for every 26 grams of protein, and three-quarters of its calories come from fat. Camembert and Edam have less: between 40 and 66 per cent of their calories are from fat. For low-fat cottage cheese, however, the figure is only about 7 per cent.

Since fats are such a concentrated form of energy (a gram of fat contains 9 calories, against the 4 calories in a gram of protein or carbohydrate), slimmers gain more by cutting out fatty foods than any others. However fat makes food palatable, giving it a good flavour and texture, so drastic reductions are not advisable. The instructions in Week One started you off on reducing the surplus fat in your diet. Here are some more relatively easy ways of cutting down:

Avoiding the hidden fat

▨ Reduce the amount of fat in the meat you eat by carefully cutting off all visible fat. Fatty meat can be recognized by the presence of marbling (streaks of white fat) running through the tissue. Avoid these cuts.

▨ As a general guide, three ounces of meat is quite enough for most adults – if you are used to larger meat portions you will probably have to increase the amount of vegetables and carbohydrate in your meals. Beans, bread, pasta, rice and even potatoes are also good sources of protein.

▨ Small quantities of fatty foods such as meat and cheese can be used to great effect by combining them with carbohydrate foods in such a way that each enhances the other. The Italians are masters of this technique – think of Bolognese sauce or Parmesan cheese with pasta. English cottage pie is another example. If you make it with a potato and cheese topping, the cheese will combine with the potato to slow down digestion and convert it into slow food.

▨ Chicken, turkey, rabbit and game are the leanest meats; young birds are leaner than old ones. Duck, goose, capon, and stewing birds are the fattest but this is nothing to worry about since you are only likely to eat them occasionally. Most of the fat in poultry lies in the skin. If you remove the skin (after cooking) you will cut your fat consumption from poultry by half.

▨ Cook roasts on a wire rack so that the fat can drain off them easily. Make the gravy from the meat juices, first discarding as much of the fat as possible. Make soup or stew ahead of time so it can be put in the refrigerator and the fat lifted off easily.

▨ Avoid milky drinks such as milky coffee or milky hot chocolate. Make these with at least half water and for the rest use semi-skimmed or skimmed milk. Some dairies will deliver semi-skimmed milk to the doorstep. St. Ivel are now selling skimmed milk called Shape in thousands of shops. Alternatively, just pour off the top of the bottle and don't shed any tears over the waste – it's bad for your heart anyway.

▨ Use low fat yoghurt with puddings instead of cream. If you want cream for a special occasion, combine it half and half with yoghurt. Avoid commercial whipped cream substitutes, which generally contain coconut oil, which is just as fattening as cream and equally bad news for the heart.

- Avocados are very high in fat. Don't think of them as vegetables – they are nearer to cheese in their fat content. Avoid whenever possible.
- Low fat spreads such as Gold or Outline can be helpful. They contain half the calories of butter or margarine.

Slimming with Eggs

Eggs are full of valuable nutrients but they also contain a lot of fat and calories. To provide a satisfying energy-balanced meal, cook them with as little fat as possible and combine them with some vegetable and carbohydrate. Unfortunately, eggs are also a major source of cholesterol – too many may contribute to heart disease. Try not to eat more than one a day. Poach or scramble eggs with milk, not butter, to avoid increasing the fat in the meal further.

Recipes

Open Sandwiches

Eggs are ideal for open sandwiches, either hard boiled or scrambled without fat in a non-stick pan.
Spread pumpernickel or Vogel's whole grain bread with curd cheese (medium fat). Combine the egg with raw vegetables and salad, smoked salmon or other smoked fish, prawns or lumpfish roe. Add a garnish of olives, radishes, fresh herbs, lemon slices or a few sunflower seeds. Instead of mayonnaise use a mixture of yoghurt and a little mustard.

Spanish Omelette

1 small onion, cut in small pieces; 1 red pepper, seeded and cut in cubes; 4oz (100-125g) cooked frozen peas or broad beans; 1 tbsp olive oil; 1 small boiled potato, cut in cubes; 1 tsp paprika; 4oz (100-125g) lean ham (optional) cut in cubes; 4 eggs; salt. For the sauce: 1lb (450g) ripe tomatoes, chopped; 1 small onion, finely chopped; chopped basil.

Heat the olive oil in a 10in (25mm) non-stick or heavy cast iron frying pan over a gentle heat. Cook the onion and the red pepper until softened, add the peas or beans and stir together until they are hot, finally stir in the cooked potato, the paprika and ham if you want it. Beat the eggs with a pinch of salt until just mixed and pour over the vegetables. Finish off under a hot grill for just long enough to set the top of the omelette. Loosen round the edge of the pan with a palette knife and turn the omelette out on to a large plate.
Serve with a fresh tomato sauce made by simmering the tomatoes and onion together until the onion is soft and the mixture is reduced. Season to taste, and stir in some basil if available.

Baked Potatoes with Eggs

4 large baking potatoes (7-8oz)(200-225g) each; 4 eggs; pepper and salt; 2oz (50g) grated cheese.

Preheat the oven to 400°F (200°C, gas mark 6). Wash the potatoes and prick them two or three times with a skewer. Bake in the hot oven for about 1 hour, or until they feel soft when pinched. Halve each potato and scoop the soft potato into a bowl. Reserve the skins. Mash the potato until fluffy and stir in the beaten yolks of four eggs and a little pepper. Beat the egg whites with a pinch of salt until stiff and carefully fold in the potato mixture using a metal spoon. Put the potato halves into a large fireproof dish and fill with the egg and potato mixture, dividing it equally between the eight shells. Sprinkle them with grated cheese and return to the oven for a further 10-12 minutes, until the tops are crispy and brown. Serve with a fairly substantial salad made with celery, apple, grated cabbage and nuts.

YOUR ABC DIARY: Week Four   Starting date:

	WALKING		JOGGING/ WALKING		SWIMMING		HOME WORKOUT	OTHER EXERCISE (e.g. cycling)
	Mins	Miles*	Mins	Miles*	Mins	Lengths	Mins	Mins
Monday								
Tuesday								
Wednesday								
Thursday								
Friday								
Saturday								
Sunday								
TOTAL								

* approximate distance, optional

ABC ROAD TEST		mins		mph				
BODY MEASUREMENTS	Date / /	Chest	Waist	Hips	Arms	Legs	Weight	

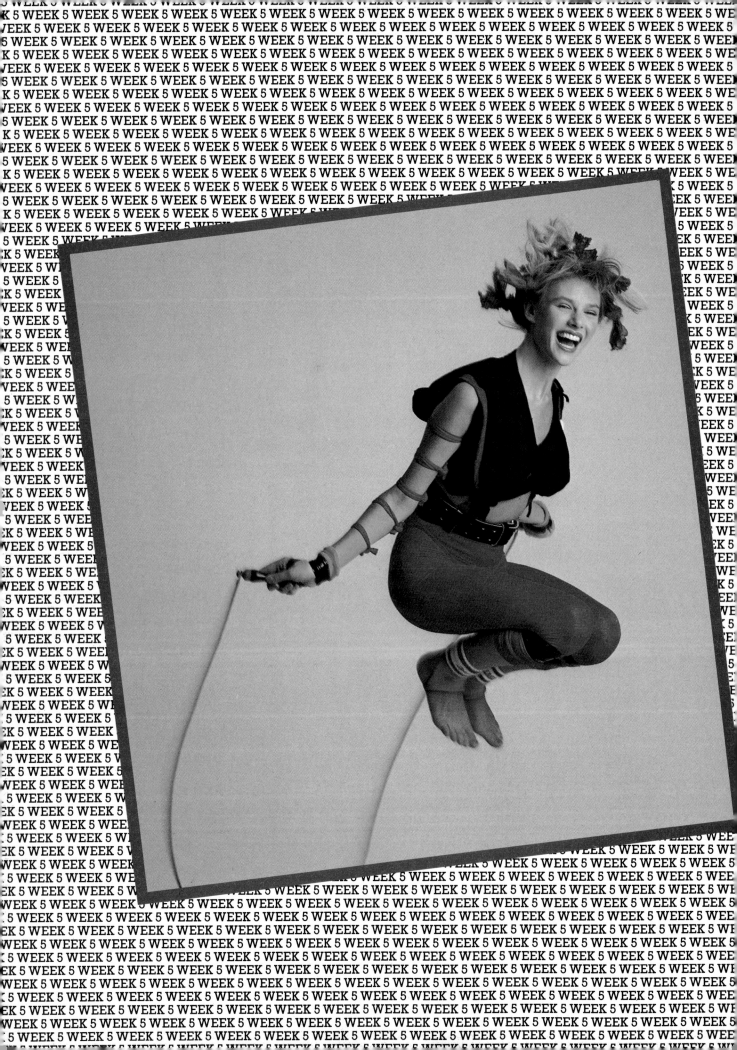

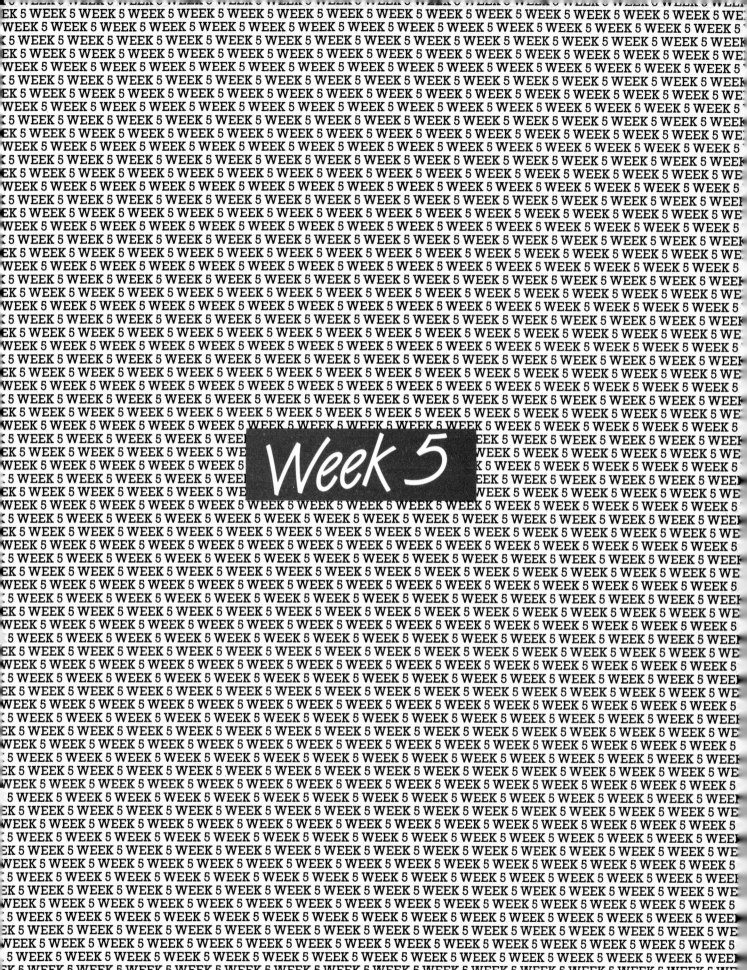

Week 5

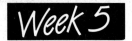

Week 5

A FOR ACTIVITY

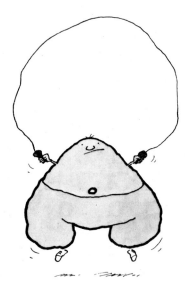

It is now time to review your progress and to see if you have any problem which is preventing you from fulfilling the exercise schedules. Look at your Diary, review your measurements, and ask yourself these questions:

1. Have you exercised for at least half an hour three times a week, except when illness or injury intervened?
Half an hour of exercise three times a week is the minimum for useful weight loss. If your Diary shows that you have not been able to fulfil this because of other commitments, then look carefully at your timetable to see how more exercise can be fitted in. This may mean giving up time in the lunch break, making better arrangements for babysitting, or changing social arrangements so that you can exercise with friends.

Don't be too discouraged if you have not yet met the minimum exercise level. It takes time and determination to change the habits of a lifetime. Congratulate yourself on what you have achieved so far and work out a practical way to do more.

If you are still not fit enough to manage the full amount of exercise, just keep going, steadily increasing the exercise you take when you can. You will obtain immediate benefits in fitness and improved sleep and some weight loss, but more dramatic weight loss will only begin when you are able to exercise more.

2. Are you pushing yourself hard enough while exercising?
It is just as well to be a bit cautious about pushing yourself at the beginning, but now you must make sure that exercise is really raising your pulse and/or increasing the speed of your breathing. If you are still not sure about this, turn back to the advice given in Week Four.

3. If your programme has been interrupted by illness or injury, have you adjusted it so you can keep going?
After a couple of days' rest, resume exercising by walking if you were previously running, or with 10 to 15 minute walks if you were doing the Walking Programme. You should be able to get to your previous level within 10 days.

If you suffered any minor injury, for example a strained ankle or knee, have you tried alternative forms of exercise, such as swimming, to keep moving until you can return to your first-choice exercise?

4. If you find it difficult to get out, have you tried the Home Workout?
There is no reason why you should not do a mixture of programmes, according to convenience and interest. You could, for example, swim once a week, walk once a week, and do the Home Workout twice a week. Progress on the swimming would of course be much slower and you would probably have to take three weeks over each of the swimming stages, but in the long term the results will be the same.

5. Have you taken steps to increase the amount of exercise in your everyday routine?
Are you, for example, walking or cycling eight minutes to the shops now instead of driving there in two when you don't have heavy shopping to carry? Are you walking for 15 minutes instead of waiting 10 minutes for a bus that gets you there in five minutes? Are you walking up and downstairs at the office or workplace instead of using the lift?
Do four or more exercise sessions this week – at least three of one type (except for Walking Programme – see below).

Walking Programme

If you have reached a walking speed of three and a half to four miles an hour and prefer to continue walking than to start jogging, take a close look at your body measurements and decide if you are satisfied with your progress. If you are not, you should increase the amount of walking you are doing or look for better ways to control your food consumption.

The best way of taking more exercise, if you are a walker, is to make your walk a daily event. You have been walking 30 to 40 minutes four days a week. Now start to take a 30 minute walk every day. Only miss a walk if you are taking some other form of exercise on that day or if you are not well. If you miss a day for some reason try to make up with a longer walk the next day.

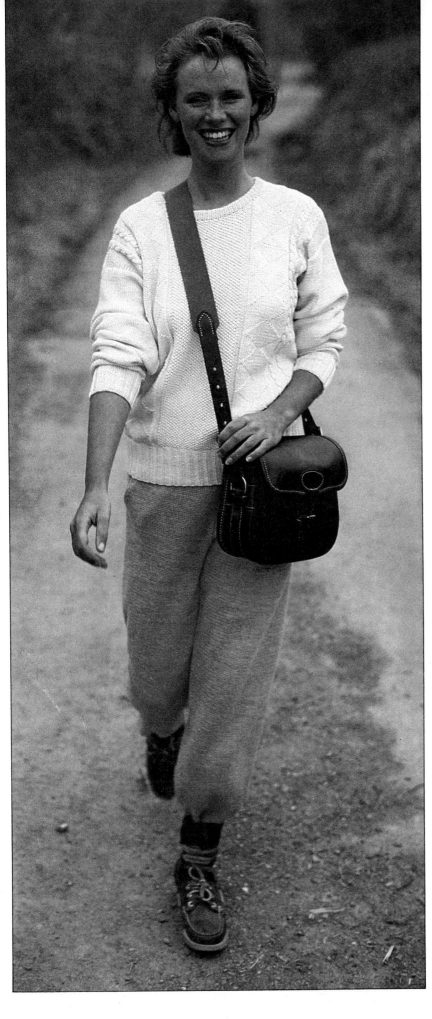

Jogging Programme

Jogging 1

■ Warm up with a brisk walk, as usual; you will know by now how long you need.

■ Jog for three minutes, walk for two minutes. Do this seven or eight times.

■ Finish with the Cool Down Stretches.

Aim gradually to increase the time you spend in continuous jogging. If two or three minutes' jogging at a time is too exhausting, continue with shorter jogs or run at a slower pace that you can sustain longer.

Jogging 2

You can now jog for between 10 and 20 minutes continuously.

■ Aim now to jog continuously for up to 25 minutes.

■ Finish with the Cool Down Stretches.

A basic principle of athletic training is to increase the stress of training, rest, then increase it again. That is more or less what you have been doing by exercising one day and resting the next. However, you can now begin to apply this principle in another way. If you have been jogging for, say, 15 minutes at a stretch and feel confident at that distance, aim now for 20 minutes or even 25. Then for the next two exercise days go back to 15 minute jogs. Then as soon as you can, repeat your 20 or 25 minute jog. Choose less hectic days for the tougher exercise, so that you have energy in reserve for your job.

ACTIVITY

Swimming Programme

Swimming 1
Warm-up

The warm up period should be used to do the Pool Exercises and improve your strokes. Practise the back crawl, perhaps, or the full backstroke (with an overhead arm movement and frogkick leg movements), swimming widths after a push-off from the side; but don't try to include these strokes in your exercise routine until you are confident that you have got them right. New strokes are not necessary for slimming purposes, but they add interest to exercising and help you to keep it up.

Exercise
- Aim to swim 16 lengths, alternating your preferred stroke with sidestroke, backstroke or another stroke.
- Repeat the Pool Exercises.
- Do the Figure Trimming Exercises.

BREATHING EXERCISES FOR SWIMMERS

These breathing exercises are for those who have not yet learnt to put their face in the water while swimming. Hold on to the rail with your hands and make the normal leg movements of breaststroke or crawl. If you are doing breaststroke, dip your face into the water and blow bubbles at the point when you would normally push your arms forward. Then lift your face out of the water, take a breath and as you kick again breathe out into the water once more. After some practice, try doing a few widths this way, blowing out into the water when you push forward and breathing in after the kick. This may be an effort at first but will eventually make swimming easier and more efficient. It will also help to eliminate neck-ache.

If you are doing crawl, breathe out into the water and turn your head to one side at the point when you would normally bring that arm out of the water. Put your face back into the water and blow out, then turn to the same side again for the next breath. After some practice, try to do a few widths in this way. You will probably find eventually that the most efficient rhythm will involve taking a breath on every other stroke of the arm on your breathing side.

Swimming 2
Warm-up

Do some short swims, a few dives and the Pool Exercises, and practise different strokes if you need to.

Exercise
- Aim to swim 24 lengths, alternating your preferred stroke and another stroke.
- Finish with the Figure Trimming Exercises.

Time test: On one of the four exercise days this week try a time test. Warm up first. Then swim for 15 minutes continuously, changing your strokes as you wish – even in mid-length if you want. Make a note in your ABC Diary of how many lengths you achieve in the time and repeat the test from time to time, perhaps once a week, to monitor your performance.

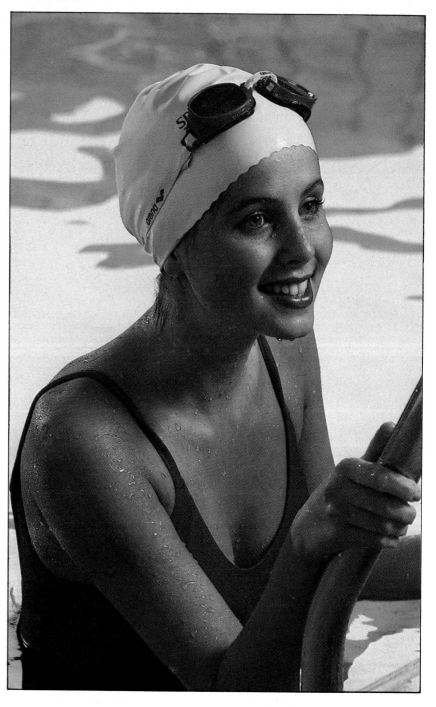

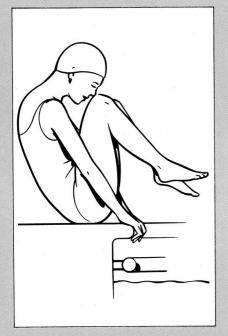

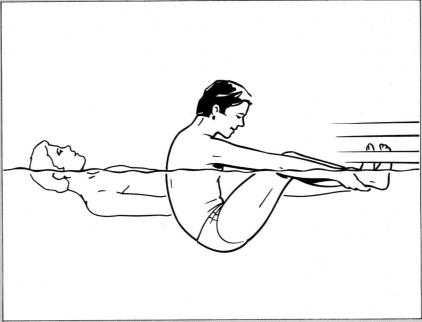

FIGURE TRIMMING EXERCISES IN THE POOL

Water provides a unique combination of resistance and buoyancy: resistance increases the effectiveness of exercises aimed at building stamina and shaping muscles, while buoyancy makes it possible to get supple with minimum wear and tear on joints, tendons and ligaments. You can make use of this in these exercises, which are designed to trim the waistline by tightening abdominal muscles.

These exercises should be done at the end of your swimming session so that they do not interrupt the aerobic sequence. Try them out at home first so that you are sure you have learnt the correct movement.

1. *Knees ups:* Sit on the edge of the pool, grip the edge and lean back slightly, pulling in your abdominal muscles. Then raise both knees towards your chest and at the same time lean forward a little to touch your knees with your head. This requires careful balance or you will fall into the pool – that is part of the challenge. Do this four times and work up to 10 times over the next few weeks.

2. *Floating sit ups:* Float on your back with your hands at your sides and, depending on the type of pool, either rest your foot on the edge of the pool or on top of the rail, pressing your heel down to grip, or hook your toes under the rail. Then bend forwards, pulling your abdomen in, and grasp your ankles for a few seconds. Do this four times in all. Build up to 20 times over a period of weeks if you can. After you have got up to 20, try doing the same exercise with hands clasped behind your head – just bending until you get into the same position as before.

3. *Waist trims:* the advantage of the water here is that it will cushion you if you find this difficult and overbalance. Stand in the shallow end and join both hands behind your head. Raise your left knee up and bring your right elbow down. Try to touch the elbow with the knee. Straighten up and do the same with the other knee and elbow. Do this four times to begin with and work up to 10 over the next few weeks.

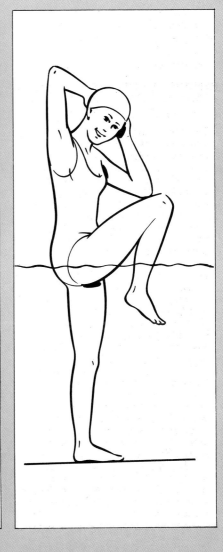

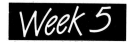

Week 5

ACTIVITY

The Home Workout

You can now begin to vary your Home Workout and spend more of your 40 minute workout doing what you enjoy most, probably dancing or room running. Whatever it is, do two sessions of at least 10 minutes each. Make certain that you are exercising vigorously enough by checking your pulse five minutes or more after starting.

If it is embarrassment at being seen jogging outside that has led you to choose home exercise, this might be a good time to think of making the break and running out of doors. By now you have built up some stamina and you know how much you can do. You could try going for a 10 minute jog, starting at your front door. All you need is some running shoes and perhaps a track suit.

Warm-up

If you would like to do something different or more energetic to music, try jumping jacks, which are a simple but vigorous exercise.

Jumping jacks: Start with your hands at your sides, legs together. Jump astride, raising your arms out to the side at shoulder level. (Avoid landing with 'knock' knees.) Jump, bringing legs together and arms to sides. Do 40 or more.

Strength-building

It is worth building up strength in the muscles of the chest and abdomen for the sake of a firmer profile and better breathing. Here are two exercises to add to your routine.

Knees-up: Sit on the edge of a chair and grip the sides with both hands. Lift one knee at a time towards your chest, leaning forwards to touch it with your head. Do this five times with each leg. Now life both together five times. Breathe out as the knees come up and in as you lower them. Stop, or go back to raising one knee at a time, if you feel any pain in your back. When you can do this without straining, gradually increase the number of repetitions to 20.

Table press-ups: These are intended for both women and men and require a solid table. Place both hands on the table, shoulder width apart. Stand far enough away to be able to lower your chest to touch the table, taking the weight on your arms and keeping your body and legs in a straight line. Breathe in as you bend your arms; breathe out as you straighten them. If this is too difficult, use a higher object. Start with four press-ups and work up to 20.

Skipping

Your ultimate goal is two five-minute sessions of 500 skips each, although you may not yet be able to manage more than two or three minutes at a time. Keep building on what you can do. Next week we suggest some rope tricks for skipping aficionados.

Stair climbing

If you continue stair climbing, increase the number of steps to between 200 and 300.

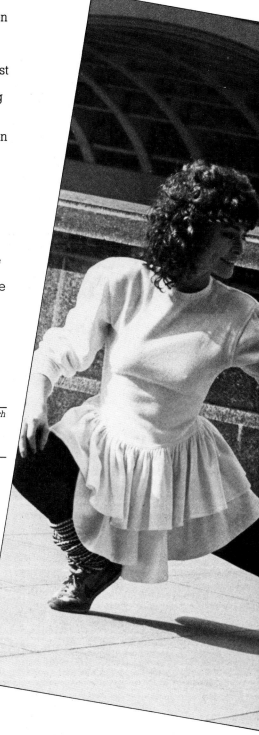

Keep-fit expert Jackie Genova limbers up in March 1983 with veteran marathon runners (from left) Roy Harris, Alexander Munro, Edward Ayling, Arthur Pigott and Madge Sharples. They were aiding The Foundation for Age Research.

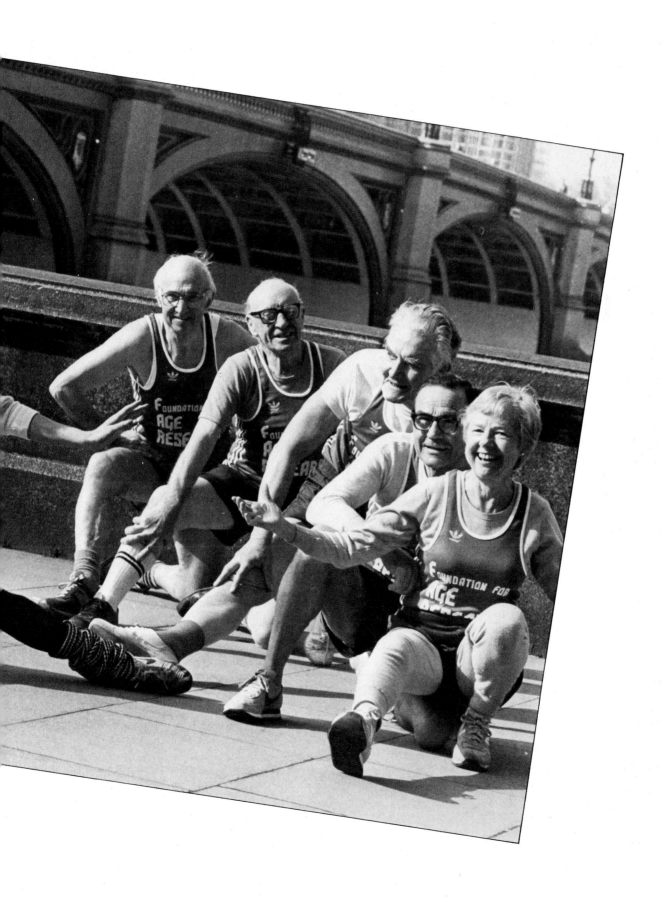

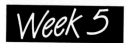

Week 5

B FOR BEHAVIOUR

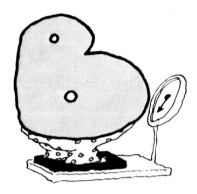

The scene: Boston, Massachusetts. Picture a man sitting down to eat his lunch. The eyes are wordly-wise, the expression firm but faintly strained. He is in his early forties, a large big-boned man. A heavy belt supports the noticeable paunch.

Before he takes the first bite, he closes his eyes. He sits there for a couple of minutes, intoning silently to himself, 'I am an adult, not a child, and I choose not to overeat.' He is an Officer of the City of Boston Police Department and his mission is to get slim.

The Power of Self-Hypnosis

This isn't the behaviour Kojak has led us to expect of cops toughened by years of duty ferreting out the criminals of urban America. But the message works. A hundred or so men attended Detective Patrick J. Brady's first course on slimming through self-hypnosis. Eighty-five lost 15 lbs or more in eight weeks, earning themselves a T-shirt bearing the legend 'City of Boston Police Department' on the front and 'Hypnosis Made Me Do It' on the back.

Eight months later, a few of the men had 'put on 3 or 4 lbs' because they had stopped using the technique, Brady concedes. 'But overall the results are looking excellent'.

Detective Brady's speciality is forensic hypnosis, on which he lectures throughout the States. He normally uses hypnosis only as an investigative tool: helping a witness in a fatal hit-and-run case to recall the licence number of the getaway car, for example. But dismay at the number of overweight policemen in Boston prompted him to put hypnosis to use in the service of slimness.

The battle against conditioning

Dependency on food is reinforced from the moment of birth, Brady points out. And people get fat because they are driven to food by childhood conditioning. 'Once you say "I am an adult, not a child", it puts you in charge,' he tells his slimmers. A man of fervent beliefs, he dismisses willpower as worthless ('When the will and the imagination are in conflict, the imagination wins every time'), has no patience for analytic delving into motives ('If you're in a swamp surrounded by alligators, you want to get out'), and will not brook half-hearted effort ('"Trying" is a word I won't tolerate because it sets people up for failure. I tell them "Either overeat, or eat like an adult, but don't just try"').

Nor does he hand out advice on diet. 'All diets work,' he says. 'It's people who don't work. I tell them they'll eat only what's good for them'.

Brady concentrates on making his subjects feel better about themselves. 'When someone needs to go on a diet, their self-image is generally poor. In hypnosis you tell them that they're good. Once you believe you're a deserving person, you'll no longer be fat,' he explains.

The negative messages directed at you when you were a child and those you now give yourself, whether you're aware of them or not, are themselves a kind of hypnosis. 'If someone tells me they can't lose weight, I tell them they've hypnotized themselves into believing they can't,' says Brady. 'It shows they're a good subject, though, and their task now is to use hypnosis to their benefit.'

Positive messages

Would-be slimmers are given a choice of positive messages (affirmations) to use during self-hypnosis, which they practise at least five times a day for two minutes each time, or even longer at first. Affirmations range in scope from the specific ('I will not eat between meals' or 'I will chew my food slowly and enjoy it more') to the general ('Overeating destroys my body and I need a healthy body to love' or 'I am an adult, not a child and I choose not to overeat') to the philosophical ('I am a good person and I will give my body the love, respect and attention it deserves').

The thought of talking to yourself in this way may strike you as bizarre. But in fact we all talk to ourselves most of the time we're awake, because it is hard for adults to think without verbalizing. And a lot of the things that people who feel unhappy about themselves say are negative. This inner dialogue plays an important part in how we evaluate ourselves and our actions, and influences our future thoughts and behaviour. Depending on its tenor, it amplifies or muffles self-esteem.

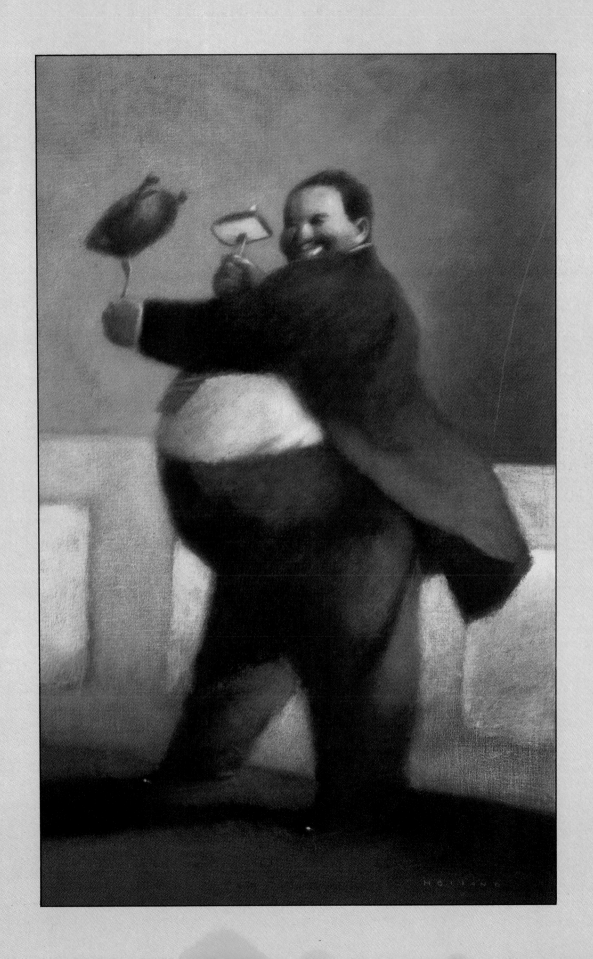

BEHAVIOUR

To benefit from positive suggestions there is no need for you to be hypnotized, so long as you are relaxed and receptive, says Dr Peter Hajek, a psychologist at the Institute of Psychiatry in London who has a special interest in hypnosis. You should be able to reach a state of mental and physical relaxation in a very short time using one of the techniques outlined last week, once the practice has become a habit.

When we're deeply relaxed, or daydreaming, or in that drowsy state between waking and sleep, the activity of our brain changes. The slower alpha wave rhythm takes over from the faster beta frequency in which we spend most of our waking lives. Beta rhythms lock us in at the level of rational thought, but alpha enables us to tap the creative capacities of our minds and put them to work for us as we choose.

In this state of heightened receptivity the subconscious is able to receive suggestions without interference from the critical, rational mind. So we can change our self-image, counteract negativity and replace self-defeating messages, thoughts and habits with more constructive ones.

These suggestions can be verbal or visual. This week we are concentrating on verbal suggestions or affirmations; next week we will cover the use of visual suggestions. Affirmations can be used to address the problem of being overweight directly. You could say to yourself, 'Taking care of my body is bringing me slimness and vitality' or, 'I am choosing to eat foods that will make me slim and healthy', for instance.

They can also address the lack of confidence and fulfilment experienced by most slimmers. 'Being fat makes people feel inadequate, second-class citizens,' says Dr Dennis Stayte, honorary secretary of the British Society of Medical and Dental Hypnosis, whose members treat many patients with weight problems by teaching them self-hypnosis. 'Lack of love in the widest sense is far and away the most common cause

SMOKING AND WEIGHT

Some smokers say that they smoke primarily because it helps to keep their weight down. When they give up smoking they put on weight. So they start to smoke again. The ABC Diet and Bodyplan can offer people with this problem new hope because the plan aims to achieve control of appetite and understanding of compulsive behaviour of which overeating is one example and smoking another.

The ABC Diet and Bodyplan can also be used by smokers who are satisfied with their weight as it is, but who fear to give up smoking because they know from experience that they will put on weight when they stop. The exercise element in the Bodyplan will enable them to eat more without putting on weight, and eventually they will probably feel able to give up smoking.

If you are a smoker you may find that you become much less interested in smoking as you become involved in the exercise part of this programme. Exercise releases natural substances in the body which give a sense of euphoria, and make it easier to do without other drugs such as tobacco or tranquillizers.

You should not attempt to give up smoking in the first half of this programme. That is expecting too much of yourself and your body. You can start now to reduce the number of cigarettes you smoke if you want to and if you can do it easily without creating a stress which makes you want to eat more.

As you approach the end of the programme you can begin to think of giving up smoking altogether. By that stage you should be taking enough exercise to have established a change in lifestyle and an interest in fitness which

will help you. If you give up and find you have an increased appetite you should be able to satisfy it with apples or fruit rather than sweets. This will limit any resulting weight gain.

If you know from past experience that it is very helpful for you to chew when you give up cigarettes then you may find nicotine chewing gum useful. This gum can be obtained from chemists on a doctor's prescription but it cannot be prescribed on the National Health Service. The gum releases nicotine – the active drug in tobacco – which is absorbed into the blood stream; this replaces the nicotine which the smoker is accustomed to getting from cigarettes. However the gum is not so satisfying to the smoker as smoking itself because the nicotine does not enter the blood stream so quickly from the mouth as it does from the lungs. It is not a miracle cure but it can be very helpful.

The health risk of smoking 20 cigarettes a day is much greater than the health risk of excess weight, except for the very small number of people who are 35 to 50 per cent overweight. To have the same risk from being overweight as smoking 20 cigarettes a day a woman 5'5" in height, whose normal acceptable weight was nine stone, would have to get up to around 13 stone – and a 5'8" man, with a normal acceptable weight of ten and half stone, would have to get to 15 stone. Looked at simply from the health point of view there is no doubt that it is best to give up smoking, even if it means putting on some weight. However, using the ABC Bodyplan you can give up smoking and minimize or avoid any weight gain.

If you are finding it difficult to give up smoking you could also try self-hypnosis (see Behaviour section this week).

of overeating. Eating is giving oneself love that is missing in other aspects of one's life,' he believes. In the course of treatment he asks his patients to imagine receiving the emotional satisfaction they feel they need. He asks them to supply their own verbal affirmations so that they will be personal and relevant. Dr Hajek notes that 'ego-strengthening suggestions can tone people up psychologically'.

How to use Positive Suggestions

1. Start recognizing the negative things you say to yourself, such as 'I can't manage on my own. I need someone to help me', 'I'm not cut out for slimming; it requires too much discipline', 'I've made a mess of things, so I may as well forget about today and start again tomorrow.'

If you can't think of any examples, play a game. Pretend you have a demon inside you whose aim is to demoralise you.

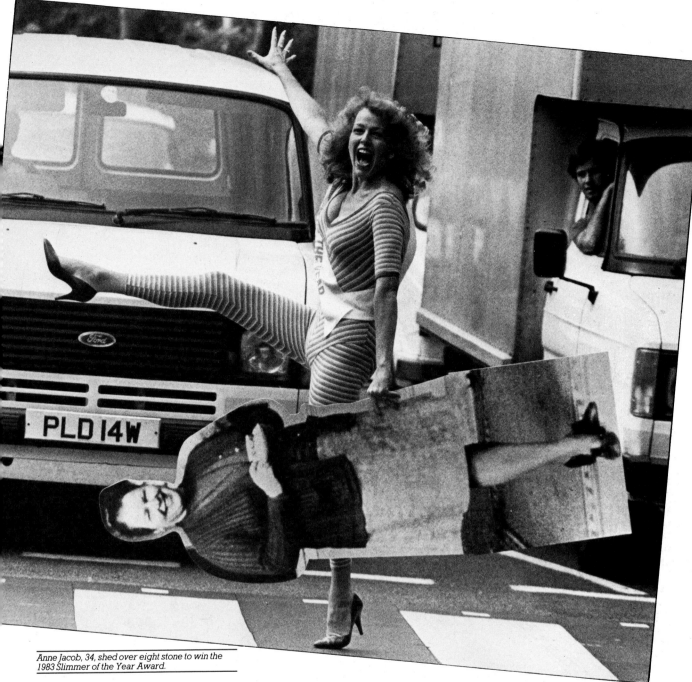

Anne Jacob, 34, shed over eight stone to win the 1983 Slimmer of the Year Award.

What does the demon say? The answers you come up with are the kind of messages you are probably using to sabotage your progress. Now let the angel inside you speak in your defence: What good things does it say? You can use these as a basis for creating your own esteem-building affirmations, which should be clear, positive, rhythmical and fairly brief. Focus on what you're aiming for, rather than what you want to avoid.

If you prefer, use some of Detective Brady's affirmations, such as 'I will chew my food slowly and enjoy it more' or 'I am a good person and I will give my body the love, respect and attention it deserves'.

2. Because being relaxed increases suggestibility, it is a good idea to give yourself positive suggestions at the end of a session of relaxation or meditation whenever possible. If you are in a hurry, try saying to yourself 'I am completely relaxed from my head to my knees to my toes' as you feel a wave of warmth and peace sweep over you from top to toe. Repeat twice. If your eyes are closed, open them, look upwards, towards your eyebrows. Hold this position until your eyelids feel heavy. Close your eyes. Now repeat two or three relevant affirmations to yourself for one minute.

3. Repeat step 2 before meals, before or during stressful situations and any time you catch yourself being unduly self-critical.

If you feel you could benefit from being hypnotized and being taught self-hypnosis by a professional, ask your doctor to contact the Secretary, The British Society for Medical and Dental Hypnosis, 42 Links Road, Ashtead, Surrey. You cannot consult a member of the society without referral from a doctor.

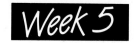

C FOR CONSUMPTION

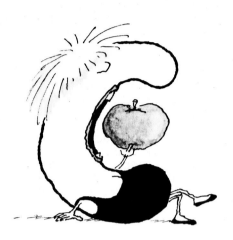

Many diets suggest reducing calories by drastically cutting carbohydrates and eating mainly meat and low energy vegetables such as lettuce, spinach or cucumber. This method of reducing weight distorts the body chemistry and can be very difficult to follow. Many people find that the shortage of carbohydrate in such diets causes feelings of hunger, tiredness or ill health.

Some of these steak-and-lettuce diets – and there are scores of them – allow unlimited fat, while others try to restrict it. But any diet that relies on red meat as a mainstay is inevitably high in fat, because red meat can contain 50 per cent or more hidden fat. The body is forced to produce energy by an incomplete process which breaks down fat in the absence of carbohydrate. As a result poisonous substances called ketone bodies are produced which give the breath a smell of acetone.

The Steak and Salad Hazard

The distortion in body chemistry produced by these diets creates a number of potential short and long term health hazards. The excessive protein puts an abnormal load on the kidneys, which have to get rid of much more nitrogenous waste material. A healthy person will have little difficulty, but anyone with weak kidneys – a not uncommon condition, especially in older people – may be harmed by the accumulation of these wastes in the blood. For example, an increase in the amount of uric acid in the blood could trigger an attack of gout in the susceptible. In the long term, these diets are dangerous because their high content of fat and cholesterol accelerates atherosclerosis and thereby increases the risk of death from heart and blood vessel disease.

Even for a few days these very low carbohydrate diets are unhealthy – people who try them often find that they feel ill, suffering from a variety of symptoms including nausea, vomiting, low blood pressure, dizziness, apathy and fatigue. The Constant Energy Diet, by contrast, is designed for maximum short term energy and long term health.

Now a husband and wife team at the Massachusetts Institute of Technology, Dr Richard and Dr Judith Wurtman, have confirmed what many dieters know – that low carbohydrate diets lead to an intense craving for carbohydrate. People on a steak-and-salad type of diet often develop such a strong desire for carbohydrate after a few days that their resolve breaks and they are driven to eat sweet snacks. Then a seesawing style of eating develops in which high protein meals which fail to satisfy hunger are followed by sweet snacks. Because the meals and snacks are nutritionally unbalanced, excessive quantities of each tend to be eaten; the would-be slimmer may fail to lose weight or may actually put it on, and, worse still, is paving the way to a bingeing problem.

Carbohydrate cravings

The Wurtmans have found that high protein meals depress the body's production of the chemical serotonin and, as a result, cause anxiety, tension or depression as well as hunger. Judith Wurtman suggests in her Carbohydrate Craver's Diet that these problems can be overcome by eating carbohydrate snacks as part of a calorie-controlled diet. She is quite content for the carbohydrate snacks she recommends to take the form of chocolate biscuits, sweets, doughnuts or sundry other empty-calorie foods.

No one takes serious issue with Dr Wurtman's brain research, although its importance for slimmers may have been exaggerated. Where her diet is contentious is in failing to draw any distinction between different types of carbohydrate, or between complex carbohydrates (whole grains, fruits, vegetables) and simple ones such as sugar.

'The brain doesn't know the difference between complex and simple carbohydrates,' says Professor Bonnie Spring of Harvard University, who has collaborated with Dr Wurtman. However, as David Jenkins' research has shown, different carbohydrates are digested at different speeds and have different effects on the blood sugar – and hence on the whole body, including the brain.

Far from assuaging carbohydrate craving, empty carbohydrates such as sweets may actually make you crave more. When Dr Martin Katahn, director of Vanderbilt University's Weight Management Programme, tested the Wurtmans' theory on 25 overweight patients, allowing them sweet snacks of 200 calories in addition to well balanced meals, six felt satisfied, two were neutral, but 17 said that the snacks made them want more.

Sugar is the most highly refined carbohydrate: it comes with no protein and no other nutrients, and in excess it disturbs normal levels of sugar in the blood and the brain. So, if you long for sweet snacks, because you have been attempting to adhere to a steak-and-lettuce diet or for some other reason, we

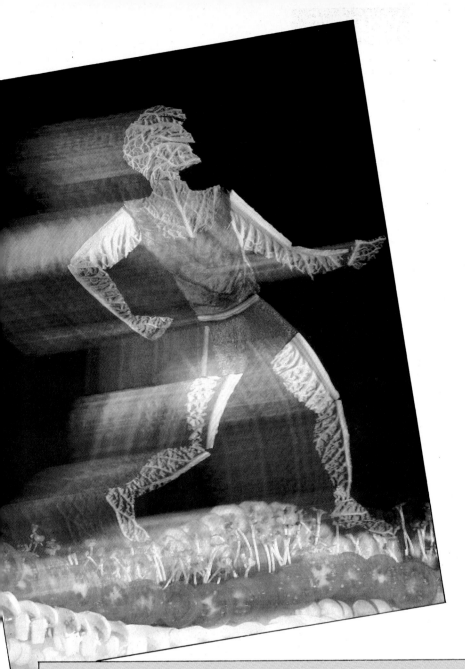

suggest you break the carbohydrate craving in another way –
by eating more slow release
carbohydrate at main meals.
▥ Cut out all heavily sweetened
foods.
▥ Cut back on meat portions if
meat has been a mainstay of
your diet.
▥ Aim to eat a slow-release
carbohydrate at each meal.
▥ Eat more vegetables.
▥ If you need a snack, eat fruit,
yoghurt, a plain biscuit or cake
made with a reduced quantity of
sugar.

FOOD AND YOUR BRAIN

More than half of the sugar circulating
in the blood is used by the brain when
the body is at rest. So when blood
sugar is low the brain cannot work
easily. The irritability, anxiety and
depression experienced by people
with low blood sugar – the condition
known as hypoglycaemia – are under-
standable symptoms of the brain
grinding slowly to a halt. If you have
ever found yourself falling asleep at the
wheel of a car and recovered after
eating a sweet biscuit then you know
what mild hypoglycaemia is.

Sweet foods which release energy
into the blood quickly bring relief for
the person who suffers from
hypoglycaemia but in the long term
this just makes the problem worse. A
vicious cycle is set up of eating sweet,
quick release foods, followed within an
hour or so by low blood sugar and
'rebound' hunger, which creates a
desire for more sweet food.

The cycle is very stressful because
when blood sugar becomes low an
emergency procedure is triggered in
the body. Adrenalin is released to
boost the sugar in the blood,
mobilizing it from the body's energy
stores. Adrenalin is the fight-or-flight
hormone, and when it is released in
this way several times a day, the result
is a feeling of physical exhaustion and
irritability.

People who are overweight often
have problems in controlling their
blood sugar. Some are prone to suffer
from hypoglycaemia: they are helped
by the Constant Energy Diet because
of the slow foods it includes in every
meal and the reduction in sugar which
it recommends.

Others who are overweight have
the opposite problem: they are unable
to clear sugar (glucose) from their
blood in the normal way. Sugar then
appears in their urine, as it does in

diabetics, although they have no other
symptoms of diabetes. This
phenomenon, known as insulin
resistance, is very common in people
who are overweight and can vary over
a wide spectrum from normal through
to diabetic.

Diabetes of this type, which does
not require insulin injections, occurs
most commonly in obese middle-aged
people and appears to be triggered by
an excessive intake of sugar and fat.
The Constant Energy Diet aims to
correct this energy imbalance, which
contributes to overweight as well as to
problems of blood sugar control.

Problems in controlling blood sugar
are also greatly relieved by exercise,
which levels out peaks and troughs in
blood sugar by training muscles to
burn fats more efficiently and making
the tissues more responsive to insulin.

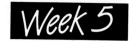

CONSUMPTION

Constant Energy Salads

Forget the feelings of starvation you have experienced while struggling to reduce weight by eating a lettuce leaf, a tomato and a slice of cucumber. Our salads are carefully balanced to provide lasting energy and variety of flavour.

Several of these salads can be served as a meal – the beans, pasta, rice and wheat are an excellent source of protein as well as slow carbohydrate. Or, if you prefer, serve them with cold meat or fish. The lighter salads can be served as a side dish to a main course or with one of the more substantial salads. Serve them with wholemeal bread, which you can use to soak up the juices if you are still hungry.

Rice Salad

8oz (225g) long grain rice, white or brown; 2oz (50g) almonds, roasted and chopped; 1oz (25g) dried apricots, chopped; 3 tbsp olive oil or sunflower oil; 1/2tsp each turmeric, ground coriander and ground cumin; 1/2 lemon, rind and juice; salt and pepper.

Roast the almonds in a medium oven until brown, chop into pieces. Soak the apricots in hot water for 10 minutes. Cook the rice, rinse and drain carefully. Put 1 tablespoon of the oil in a large heavy pan and heat it gently, add the spices and cook for a moment or two, stirring well. Remove from the heat. Drain the apricots and add these to the pan, together with the remaining ingredients. Stir well until the rice is evenly coloured. Put the rice in a dish and serve at room temperature. (If the rice has to be refrigerated, allow it to return to room temperature before serving.)

Broccoli Salad

1lb(450g) broccoli, trimmed; 2 sweet red peppers. For the sauce: 1 clove garlic; 1 tbsp olive or sunflower oil; 8oz (225g) tomatoes, chopped; salt and pepper.

Cook the broccoli until just tender, rinse with cold water and drain well. Cut the broccoli lengthways into smaller pieces. Grill the red peppers, turning them as they brown. Wrap them in a clean cloth and allow them to cool for 10 minutes. Peel off the wrinkled skin and slice the peppers into thin strips, removing the seeds and the inner membranes.

Cook the crushed garlic in the oil until just beginning to brown, add the chopped tomatoes and season with salt and pepper. Simmer gently for 5 minutes or so. Remove from the heat and liquidize, process or press through a sieve. Arrange the broccoli in a flat serving dish, pour the sauce over it and arrange the strips of red peppers round the edge.

The red peppers can be finely chopped instead of grilled, but this method adds a subtle smoky flavour to the salad. Other vegetables – courgettes, green beans or cauliflower – can be used instead of broccoli.

Fish Salad

This makes a very pretty light luncheon or supper dish. If mussels are out of season, or if you dislike them, prawns can be used instead.

8oz (225g) mussels, in their shells, washed and scrubbed; 4 scallops; 8oz (225g) firm white fish (turbot, halibut, brill); 12oz (350g) small new potatoes, scrubbed; 1lb (450g) fresh broad beans or 8oz (225g) frozen broad beans; 1 glass white wine; 1 bay leaf; 4 peppercorns. For the dressing: 3 tbsp yoghurt; 2 tbsp double cream; 2 tbsp fish stock; 1/2 tsp mild curry powder; salt (optional).

Put the mussels in a shallow pan with the wine, bay leaf and peppercorns over a fairly high heat. Shake the pan and remove the mussels to a plate as they open. Strain the cooking liquid into a jug and make it up to 1/2 pint (300ml) with water. Return this liquid to the rinsed pan (it probably won't need any salt) and gently poach the fish for 5-10 minutes – the cooking time will depend on the thickness of the piece. If the liquid doesn't cover the fish, turn it over half way through the cooking. Remove from the pan and allow to cool. Cut the white part of the scallops in half horizontally and poach in the cooking liquid for 3 or 4 minutes, adding the coral (the bright orange part of the scallop) for the last 2 minutes. Remove the scallops from the pan and reserve the cooking liquid. Boil it hard until reduced by about one third.

Cook the potatoes in their skins, allow to cool and cut into halves, or quarters if they are too large. Cook the broad beans until just tender. Take the mussels from their shells, flake the fish and arrange all the ingredients in a shallow serving dish, using the mussels and scallops for decoration. Mix the ingredients for the dressing, tasting it to see if it needs any salt added. Pour it over the salad and leave to stand at room temperature for a while before serving.

Pasta Salad

6oz (175g) pasta shells or penne; 6oz (175g) cold chicken or turkey; 6oz (175g) French beans; 2 hard-boiled egg whites, chopped. For the dressing: 3 tbsp Dijon mustard; 2 hard-boiled egg yolks, mashed; salt and pepper; 4 tbsp olive or sunflower oil; 2 tbsp yoghurt; 2 tbsp chopped gherkin pickles; 2 tbsp chopped capers; chopped parsley.

Cook the pasta in plenty of boiling salted water until just done. Drain, rinse in cold water and drain again well. Chop the chicken or turkey into pieces roughly the same size as the pasta. Cook the beans and cut each one into three or four pieces. Combine these ingredients with the chopped egg whites.

For the dressing, mix the mustard with the egg yolks and add salt and pepper. Stir in the oil, a few drops at a time, as when making a mayonnaise. Finally, stir in the yoghurt and the finely chopped pickles and capers. Mix this dressing into the salad and sprinkle with a little parsley.

This is a good light lunch or supper dish served with a green salad. Cooked broad beans may be used instead of the French beans.

Three Bean Salad

The beans should be soaked separately in the normal way and drained well. If using tinned beans, drain, rinse and drain again.

8oz (225g) cooked flageolet beans, or one 14oz (400g) tin; 8oz (225g) cooked red kidney beans or one 14oz (400g) tin; 8oz (225g) cooked butter beans or one 14oz (400g) tin. For the dressing: 1 tbsp lemon juice; 3 tbsp olive or sunflower oil; 2fl oz (50ml) tomato juice; salt and pepper; 6 sage leaves, chopped.

Mix the beans together. Make a dressing with the lemon juice, oil and tomato juice, season and add the sage. Pour over the beans, mix and leave to stand at room temperature for an hour or two before serving.

This is a good salad to serve at a buffet supper; it is sustaining and looks very colourful.

Winter Salad

8oz (225g) celery; 2 red eating apples; 4oz (100-125g) button mushrooms; 3oz (75g) shelled walnut halves. For the dressing: 4 tbsp walnut, olive or sunflower oil; 2 tsp French mustard; 1 tbsp white wine vinegar; salt and pepper.

Chop the celery, apples and mushrooms so that all the pieces are roughly the same size, and put into a bowl with the walnut halves. Stir in the dressing, made by mixing the oil into the mustard then adding salt, pepper and finally the vinegar. Serve with warm pitta bread and cheese or lean cold meat.

Tabbouleh (Cracked Wheat Salad)

This recipe uses burghul or pourgouri, a form of cracked wheat that has been hulled and parboiled, so it is not necessary to cook it, It is found in many Greek and Middle Eastern stores.

4oz (100-125g) burghal or pourgouri; 6 medium size tomatoes, chopped; 6 spring onions, finely sliced; 1 bunch parsley, chopped; 1 bunch of mint or fresh coriander, chopped (optional). For the dressing: 4 tbsp lemon juice; 4 tbsp olive or sunflower oil; salt and pepper.

Soak the burghul in plenty of cold water for 10 minutes. Drain in a colander lined with a clean dry teatowel; when most of the water has drained away squeeze out the rest by wringing the cloth hard. Put the burghal in a serving dish and add the tomatoes, spring onions, parsley, and either mint or coriander if you like the taste and can find it easily. Pour on the lemon juice and oil, season with salt and pepper and stir well. This makes a very good accompaniment to grilled chicken or kebabs. In the Middle East they scoop up the *tabbouleh* with small vine leaves; the leaves from a crisp cos lettuce would do instead.

Chicory, Orange and Watercress Salad

2 or 3 heads of chicory; 2 large oranges; 1 bunch watercress, washed and trimmed; 2 tbsp olive oil; salt and freshly ground black pepper.

Trim the chicory, separate the leaves (it is not usually necessary to wash them), and arrange them in a dish. Peel the oranges, removing the pith and inner skin, and cut them into segments or rings, catching as much juice as possible. Add the orange and juice to the chicory. Just before serving add the watercress to the salad and trickle over it the olive oil and some salt and black pepper. This makes a very good salad to serve with roast meat or game.

Cole Slaw

This recipe makes a filling salad. The tofu should be available from health food stores; it is made from soy milk, is low in calories and fat, but has a high protein content. It makes a very good low-fat mayonnaise substitute. A spoonful of Dijon mustard is a good addition if you like a sharper dressing.

12oz (350g) white cabbage, weighed after trimming outer leaves and stalk; 1 large carrot; 1 tbsp caraway seeds (optional). For the dressing: 8oz (225g) tofu; 3 tbsp olive or sunflower oil; 2 tbsp lemon juice; 2 tbsp tomato juice; salt and pepper.

Slice the cabbage as finely as possible (some food processors have a special blade for this purpose). Scrub the carrot clean, grate it finely and combine with the cabbage, stirring in the caraway seeds if you like them. To make the dressing, put all the ingredients in a liquidizer and process until creamy. Mix into the salad, check the seasoning and allow to marinate for a while before serving.

Variation: Red cole slaw. Substitute red cabbage for white and use a grated apple instead of a carrot. Use 2 tablespoons of apple juice instead of tomato juice in the dressing.

HOW TO COOK BEANS

This method is recommended by Elizabeth David in *French Provincial Cooking*; it removes the oxide of potassium and makes the beans more digestible. It reduces the cooking time considerably which is also an advantage.
1. Wash the beans carefully and remove any foreign bodies.
2. Bring the beans to the boil in water (1 pint for each 4 oz. of dried beans), add no salt at this stage, simmer for 1 minute, cover and remove from the heat. Allow to soak for 40 minutes, longer if you like.
3. Drain the beans; running the cold tap while doing this will help to get rid of the unpleasant smell.
4. Return the beans to the saucepan, cover with plenty of cold water and simmer until done. If using the pressure cooker make sure that it is not more than one third full. Add salt for the last 5 minutes of the cooking time. If it is added earlier it will toughen the beans.
5. Beans are at their freshest in the autumn and need least cooking then; as the year advances the beans become older and tougher and need more cooking.
6. It is extremely difficult to give accurate times for cooking beans – so much depends on the age, growing conditions and harvesting of the beans. However, as a rough guide the following times may be helpful. Soak the beans as suggested above.

Haricots
Simmer for approximately 1 hour. Pressure cooker: 8 minutes at high pressure.
Flageolets (Green haricots)
Simmer for approximately 1 hour. Pressure cooker: 8 minutes at high pressure.
Red kidney beans
Simmer for approximately $1\frac{1}{4}$ hours. Pressure cooker: 10 minutes at high pressure. (It is very important that these beans are well cooked or they will cause unpleasant stomach upsets. Be sure also to throw away the cooking water which contains the substance responsible for this.)
Butter beans
Simmer for 45 minutes. Pressure cooker: 6 minutes at high pressure.
Chick peas
Simmer the chick peas for 2 or 3 minutes before soaking, or soak in cold water overnight. Simmer for 1 hour or more. Pressure cooker: 10-15 minutes. If the chick peas are still not done continue to cook them in the pan until soft.

YOUR ABC DIARY: Week Six					Starting date:			
	WALKING		JOGGING/ WALKING		SWIMMING		HOME WORKOUT	OTHER EXERCISE (e.g. cycling)
	Mins	Miles*	Mins	Miles*	Mins	Lengths	Mins	Mins
Monday								
Tuesday								
Wednesday								
Thursday								
Friday								
Saturday								
Sunday								
TOTAL								

* approximate distance, optional

ABC ROAD TEST	mins	mph	SWIMMING TIME TEST	lengths	mins

BODY MEASUREMENTS	Date / /	Chest	Waist	Hips	Arms	Legs	Weight

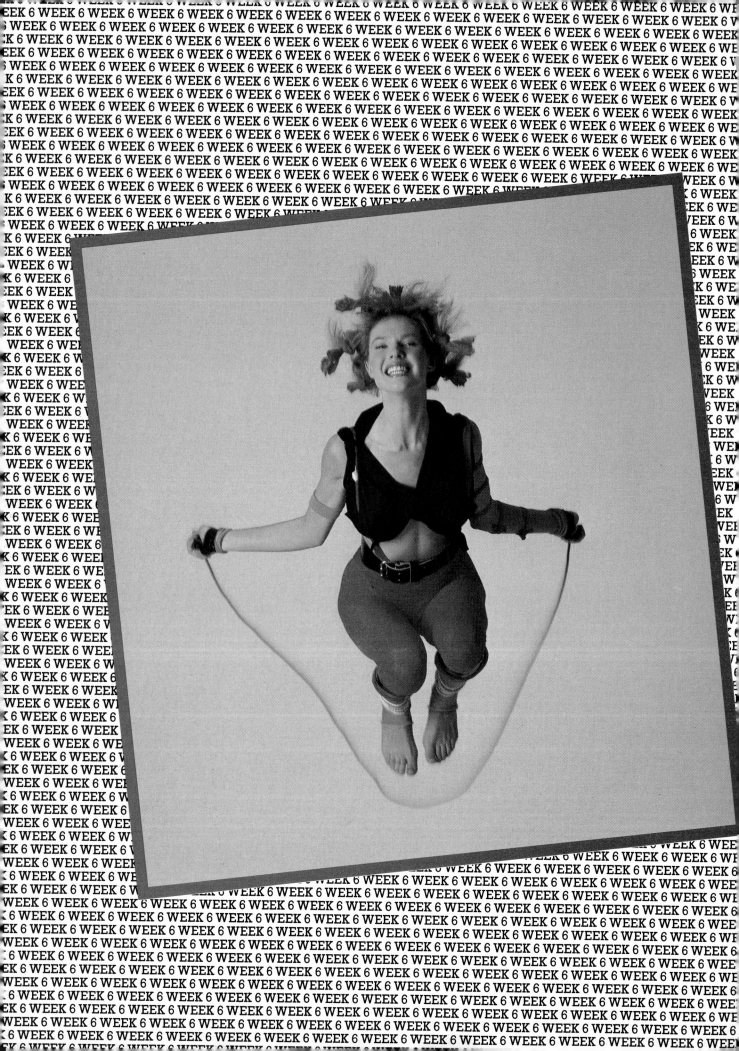

Week 6

A FOR ACTIVITY

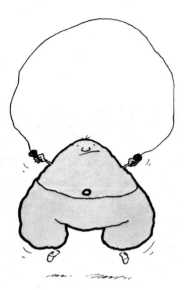

Congratulations on reaching Week Six of your exercise plan. The first five weeks are the toughest.

If you have been unable to keep up, do not feel you have failed. Continue to work steadily at your own pace. It is a considerable achievement to have stuck with the plan for five weeks, whatever level you have reached. If you have fallen behind because you are exercising only sporadically, concentrate your efforts on setting up a regular routine – intermittent exercise brings little improvement in fitness.

Do four or more exercise sessions this week – at least three of one type (except for Walking Programme – see below).

Walking Programme

Walk briskly for 30 to 40 minutes at least five times a week.
All the walking you have done in the past weeks will have strengthened your leg muscles. For all-round development, you should now add some exercise to strengthen your abdominals and upper body. Spend a few minutes doing the knees-up exercise and table press-ups described in the Home Workout in Week Five. These will not help you to slim and are not a substitute for walking, but they will improve your figure and posture. The press-ups strengthen arms, chest and shoulders. The knees-ups do the same, as well as tightening the abdominals and increasing flexibility in the spine. Start with five repetitions of each exercise and build up to 20.

Jogging Programme

Jogging 1
▨ Start with your usual warm up.
▨ Run for three to five minutes and walk for about two minutes. Repeat for 20 to 30 minutes.
▨ Walk for at least five minutes to cool off.
▨ Finish with the Cool Down Stretches.
Your aim now should be to find a comfortable pace that doesn't make you stop for breath and that you could keep up more or less indefinitely (but don't try just yet).

Jogging 2
▨ Warm up as usual.
▨ Jog for 20 minutes.
▨ Walk briskly for 10 to 15 minutes.
▨ Walk for five minutes to cool down.
▨ Finish with the Cool Down Stretches.
You can begin to introduce greater variety into your jogging in one of two ways – by finding more varied terrain, including some hills, or by varying the speeds at which you run.

Hill training: this helps to build stamina and increase speed.

Running uphill strengthens muscles, and running downhill lengthens the stride. After warming up, you should always run for five minutes on the flat before attempting a hill. Short, steep hills are best tackled fast – sprint up them if you can, springing with the legs and pumping with the arms. At the top, try to keep jogging, but slowly, until you get your breath back. Long, gentle hills, which can be the worst, should be tackled more sedately. Be prepared to slow down to a walk if the effort is too great.
    If you have been running mostly on roads, try to get to a large park or to the country once a week to get the feel of wide open spaces.

Fartlek (Swedish for 'speed play') involves speeding up the pace of running for short intervals. Fartlek can be used to make a workout tougher and less repetitive. Athletes may aim to make half their workout really tough running by introducing bursts of speed; this is too strenuous for the non-competitive runner. But you can enjoy the playful spirit of *fartlek* by running fast (though not too fast) for short distances of say 100 or 200 yards. Don't aim for fixed intervals: just speed up as the spirit takes you, no more than two or three times at first, returning to your normal slow-to-medium pace afterwards. Consciously relax your body after a speed burst.

Swimming Programme

Swimming 1
▨ Warm up for a few minutes.
▨ Do the Pool Exercises.
▨ Swim 18 lengths, resting briefly every four lengths if you want to.
▨ Repeat the Pool Exercises.
▨ Finish with the Figure Trimming Exercises.

Swimming 2
▨ Aim to swim 28 lengths. Vary the strokes to keep up a good pace without tiring and rest briefly after six or eight lengths if you need to.
▨ Finish with the Figure Trimming Exercises.

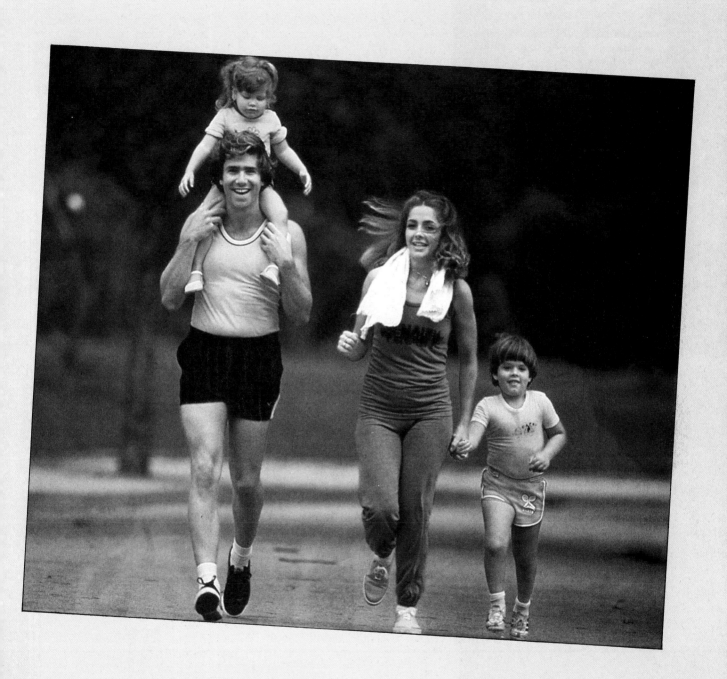

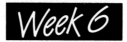

ACTIVITY

The Home Workout

If you continue with the Home Workout at this level you should be able to slim steadily. But we suggest you join an aerobics or keep-fit class so that, once a week at least, you bolster your motivation, meet people who share your interests and learn new moves or exercises that you can incorporate into your routine. Now that you are so much fitter, you must work harder to get your pulse up to the training level. If you're in doubt about whether a workout is vigorous enough for you, check your heart rate.

Skipping: Rope Tricks

There is nothing better than two-step skipping for losing weight – but these additional steps make skipping more fun.

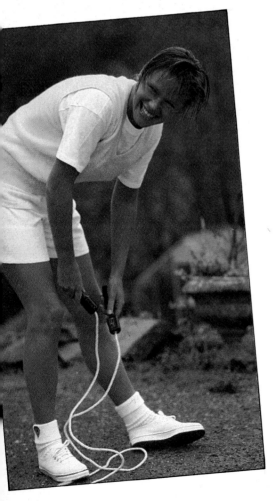

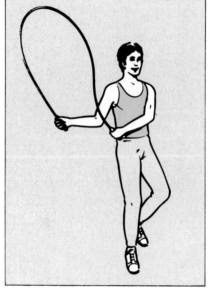

The matador jump: children do this one to the rhythm 'one, two, three i-ena, four five, six i-ena', etc. Bobby Hinds, the doyen of skipping, calls it the matador jump. Begin by doing it to the ordinary skipping step (feet together) then, when you have mastered it, to the two-step. Bring the rope over your head, then, with both hands to one side, swing the rope round once outside the body. Swing the rope up behind your head, bring it down again and jump through it once more.

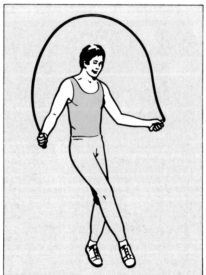

Leg cross-overs: Skip by jumping up and down on one leg, then the other. When you have got into the rhythm, cross the 'resting' leg in front and lightly touch the ground

on the other side with the toe. Bring the leg back and touch again. Continue crossing the leg back and forth to the rhythm. Repeat with the other leg. This is a great challenge to co-ordination and will take a lot of practice.

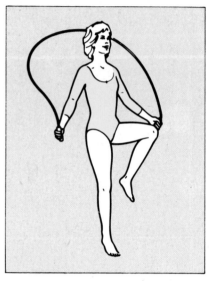

High-step two-step: This exercise is first-class for strengthening abdominal muscles. Jump twice on the left foot then twice on the right. Before switching, lift the right leg high in front. As a variation you can jump five or 10 times on each leg before changing.

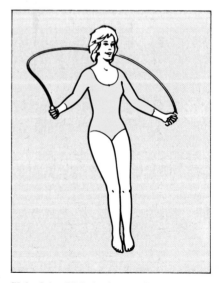

Ski-skip: This imitates the movement made by downhill skiers and calls for balance, co-ordination and muscular strength. Skip with the legs together, jumping to left and right of centre.

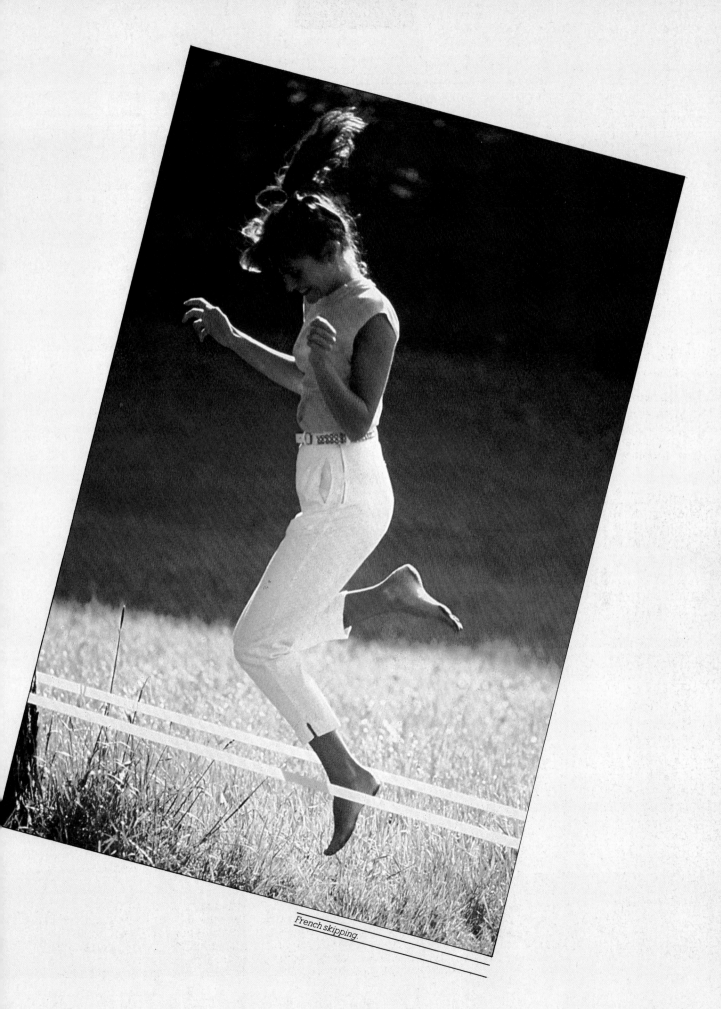

French skipping.

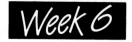

B FOR BEHAVIOUR

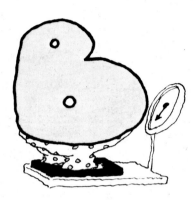

Cast your eye over Rubens' goddesses in The Judgement of Paris and your reaction, especially if you're a woman, is likely to be one of distaste or even revulsion. These cellulite-ridden Olympians may have embodied the ideal of feminine beauty in Rubens' time, but today we value a leaner look. Jane Fonda, with her long, sinewy limbs and firm muscles, is the icon of the Eighties.

The way we want to look is dictated by culture, not nature, and cultural norms are fickle and arbitrary, as well as tyrannical. Women have traditionally been prepared to distort their physiology in pursuit of fashion – think of the Victorians' corsets, which displaced internal organs for the sake of an 18-inch waist, or flappers in the Twenties bandaging their breasts to achieve a boyish outline. Since the Second World War alone, women have sought to emulate figures as diverse as Jane Russell, Twiggy and Bo Derek.

There have always been stereotypes of physical attractiveness, of course, to which women did their best to conform, but probably never before has dissatisfaction with the female form been so widespread, because social standards and media bombardment with images of desirability have combined to shape the expectations of millions of women. Commercials, fashion magazines, girlie magazines, and now physical fitness magazines and videos tell women what to look like. Inevitably, most fall short.

Even the most attractive models and performers are only too ready to catalogue their physical shortcomings, focussing obsessively on minute details of shape. These revelations may make riveting reading for slimmers whose defects are more readily discernible, but they point to a disturbing and almost universal lack of acceptance by many people of their own body.

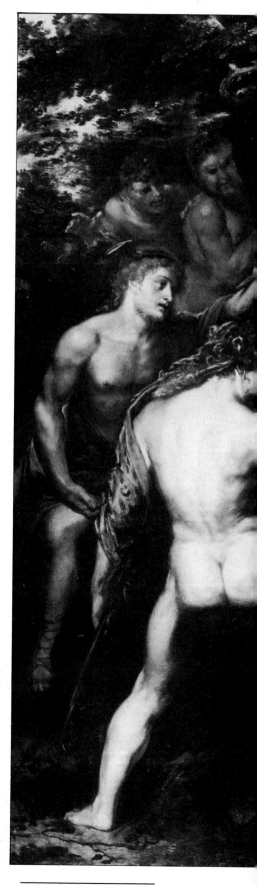

Rubens' 'The Judgement of Paris'.

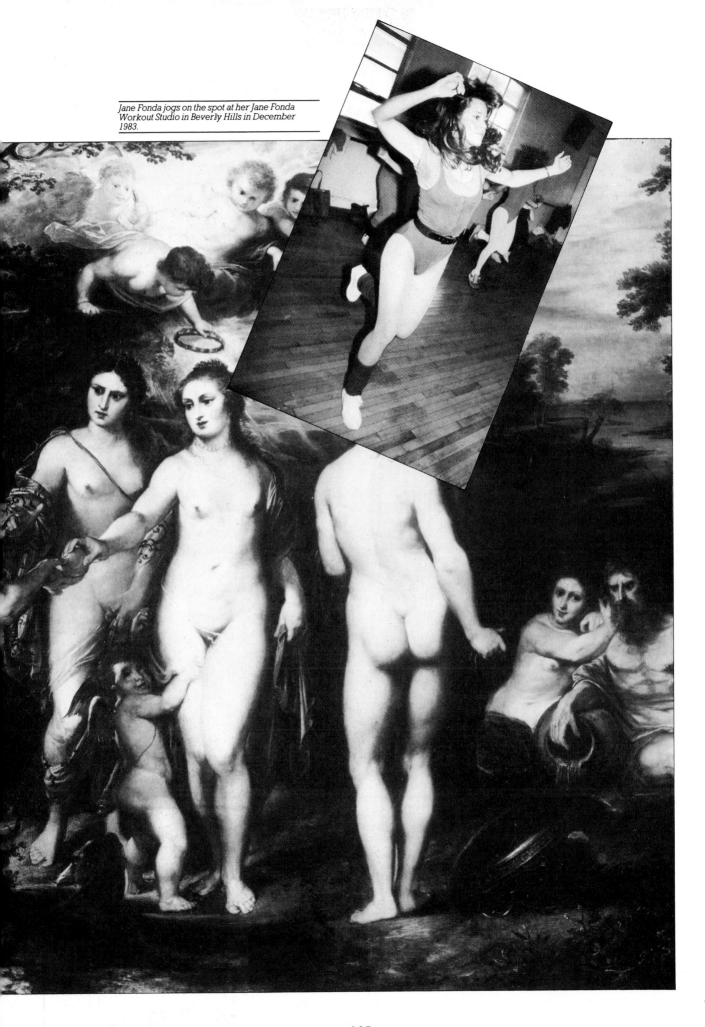

Jane Fonda jogs on the spot at her Jane Fonda Workout Studio in Beverly Hills in December 1983.

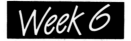

Week 6

B E H A V I O U R

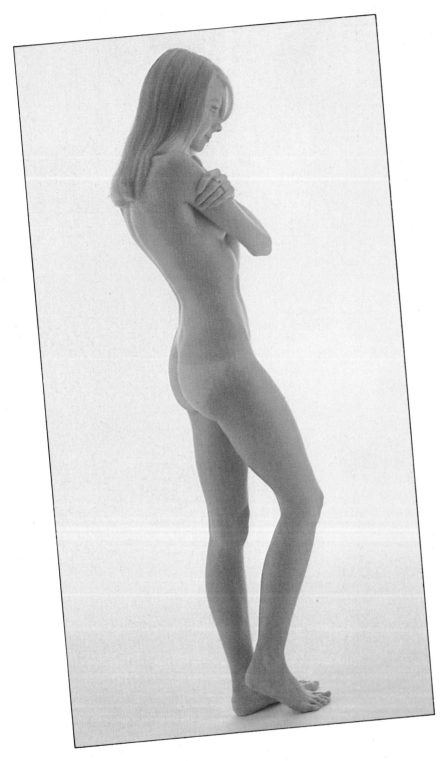

Is your Image of Yourself Disturbed?

The image we have of our body is important because it is so closely linked to how we feel about ourselves as people. In a society that views fatness as ugly, it takes a lot of strength to feel good about yourself if you are large, particularly at adolescence, when hormonal changes occur and body image is consolidated.

Anyone who has a problem with their weight or with eating is likely to have a poor or distorted body image. Bingers, people who have lost a lot of weight, and anorexics are notoriously unable to estimate their size correctly.

'Being fat in our society is such a stigma that people who are fat develop a distorted body image,' says Celia McCrea, a clinical psychologist at Queen's University, Belfast, who has been treating women with disturbances of body image and resistant weight problems. 'This may in turn predispose them to depression and to not taking the usual care of themselves. The problem is circular. Esteem-lowering experiences feed the distorted body image and lead to overeating as well as to guilt and shame.'

Learning to accept your body the way it is constitutes an important step that increases your self-esteem generally. Being able to see your body as a thing of beauty in its own right, without reference to other people's arbitrary stereotypes, is a liberating experience. This doesn't happen overnight, of course, and it doesn't mean that you will no longer want to change your body. It means that you will be relieved of the negative messages and despair that stop so many people from achieving long-term change. A better body image can also help you lose weight.

The women who took part in Celia McCrea's 20-week study found that by getting used to seeing themselves on video they became less disturbed by their appearance. 'Now they have a new inner acceptance. They're

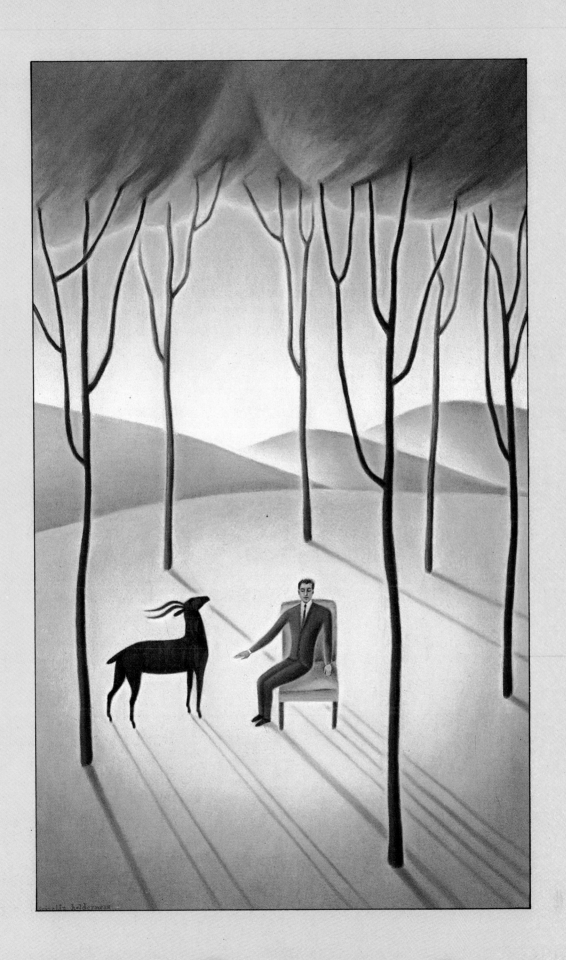

B E H A V I O U R

able to take responsibility for themselves instead of expecting some sort of magic from a doctor or therapist.'

This new self-acceptance helped to produce weight loss. Of the 12 women in the study, two got dramatically slimmer, eight lost a little. A similar experience has been reported by many women who have taken part in the groups for compulsive eaters run by Susie Orbach (of *Fat is a Feminist Issue* fame) and others at the Women's Therapy Centre in London. The women who attend these groups commonly find that when they start to accept their bodies the way they are, for all their size, they start to lose weight naturally, without trying.

Here is a four-point plan for improving body image.

1. Accept yourself

The more you accept your body the way it currently is, the easier, paradoxically, you will find it to change. The more you reject and deny yourself as your are – your body, your looks in general, yourself as a whole – the more energy will be tied up in that denial.

Learn to observe without judging. Look at yourself in a full-length mirror, preferably naked. Notice the contours of your body, the curves and bumps, the colour and texture of the skin, how the different parts relate to each other. Being able to do this without grimacing or wincing at what you see is an important step in the right direction. If you find this exercise disturbing, do it with your clothes on until you feel more comfortable. Watch yourself walking about, too. This is how the rest of the world sees you most of the time.

Do not be tempted to go on a crash diet. Distortions in perception of body size are more likely to be triggered by rapid changes in weight. Anorexics who gain weight slowly are more successful in keeping it on than those who gain it fast. For fat people, fast weight loss is a psychological shock akin to losing a limb; the body image does not get a chance to adjust to the new body reality. They often cling to a fat 'phantom body size', especially if they have been overweight

since adolescence. Slow loss makes adjustment easier.

2. Keep moving

Exercise is one of the best ways of improving body image and has the capacity to make you feel better about your body as well as directly improving its shape. It enhances overall self-confidence and relieves anxiety and depression, and it gives you a greater feeling of control, because you come to perceive your body as an active instrument rather than just a passive object for others' appraisal.

3. Picture yourself changing

Body image is one of the functions directed by the right side of the brain, the half that works in images and symbols and is the seat of the emotions. (The left side, which is the seat of reason and logic, works with language, numbers and sequences.) Logic makes little impact on body image, but a technique that can have powerful effect on it is creative imagery, or visualization, in which you purposefully direct your mental pictures. It works because it is a right-brain activity that sidesteps the rational mind, tapping the source from which intuition, creativity and imagination flow.

A simple exercise designed to improve body image using this technique is given in the section All in the Mind's Eye. Practise it regularly after relaxation or meditation. You will find that it not only enhances your body image but actually speeds up weight loss and change in shape, because the body responds to what the mind visualizes. If you think this sounds fanciful, you should know that creative imagery has been found very helpful in treating the sick. Dr Carl Simonton, a physician specializing in cancer, and his wife, psychotherapist Stephanie Matthews-Simonton, have shown in their research in Texas that cancer patients can improve their response to treatment by visualizing the destruction of their cancer cells during regular periods of creative imagery. The technique is also being used successfully by athletes in several countries to enhance their performance.

4. Know yourself

Exploring the meanings that you have attached to your body size is an important step towards improved body image. These meanings are different for everyone. Being large (or larger than you think you would like to be) can be connected with feelings of vulnerability or protection, self-sufficiency or dependency, power or lack of control. 'Being fat can be a coping mechanism to avoid other problems of living,' according to Celia McCrea, who encourages her patients to become aware of their fears of becoming slim and the advantages they gain from being overweight.

Start noticing the feelings and associations attached to your weight. Do not judge them. Observe them as objectively as you can and write them down, if you wish, as a way of keeping in touch with yourself. Next week we give more help in finding some of the personal meanings you may have attached to your weight.

All in the Mind's Eye

This exercise in creative imagery is designed to help you to change your body and to think better of it. It should be practised in a relaxed state, ideally after deep relaxation or meditation.

■ Sit comfortably in a darkened, quiet room, and say to yourself as you exhale, 'I am completely relaxed from my head to my knees to my toes'. As you say this, feel a wave of warmth and relaxation sweep over you from head to toe. Repeat twice.

■ Eyelids closed, roll your eyes upwards until your eyes and lids feel tired and heavy.

■ Draw a picture in your mind's eye of an ideal setting, real or imagined. The choice is yours. It can be a tropical beach, a glade in a forest, a mountain valley or a peaceful lake. Bring all your senses into play. See the landscape in vivid detail – the shapes, colours and textures. See the ground, the sky, the vegetation, the wildlife. Feel the sun. Feel the air against your skin. If there is water in your scene, hear the noise it makes. Put your hand in the water and notice the feel. What smells do you detect? Bring the picture to life as vividly as you can.

■ Now clearly place yourself in the setting. See or feel yourself in relation to the landscape. Move about; see yourself as you want to be – slim, supple, fit, moving freely, feeling good about yourself. Bend over to touch the ground. Notice how easy your movements are. Picture the clothes you are wearing in detail. Notice how they are comfortable and make you feel good. Notice your limbs are shapely, your skin is smooth and firm, your eyes sparkle. You give off a glow of health and well-being.

■ See yourself slowly walking out of the picture, in a relaxed, confident way.

■ Sit still for a couple of minutes before bringing your attention back into the room. Do not rush.

■ Refer to that image of confidence and well-being at regular intervals. Make it part of your pictorial repertoire. Return to your ideal setting any time you want to relax or give yourself a boost.

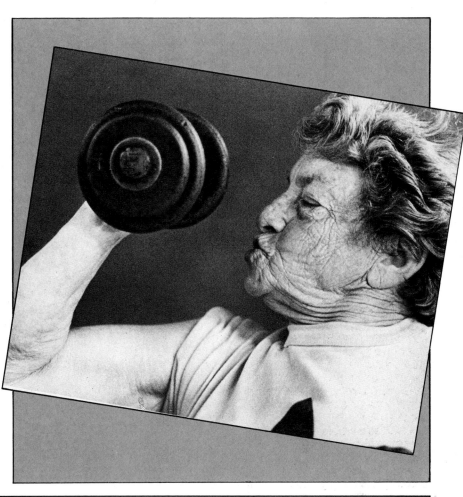

BODY IMAGE QUESTIONNAIRE

Rate yourself on each of the statements below, rating 0 if it is never applicable, 1 if it is occasionally true for you, 2 for sometimes and 3 for frequently.

I dislike seeing myself
in mirrors 0 1 2 3

Shopping for clothes can be uncomfortable because it makes me more aware of
my size and shape 0 1 2 3

I think my body is ugly 0 1 2 3

I avoid exercising in public
because of my appearance .. 0 1 2 3

I feel embarrassed about my appearance in front of someone of the opposite
sex 0 1 2 3

Certain parts of my body are OK, but the overall
effect is not 0 1 2 3

I'm ashamed to be seen in public in a bikini, swimsuit
or shorts.............................. 0 1 2 3

I compare myself with other people to see if they
are fatter than I am 0 1 2 3

I feel that other people must think my body is
unattractive......................... 0 1 2 3

I may joke about my appearance but I'm very sensitive if other people
remark on it 0 1 2 3

I feel guilty about my size ... 0 1 2 3

I don't like having my
photograph taken............... 0 1 2 3

I spend a lot of time thinking about my
appearance 0 1 2 3

If I were slimmer I think I would be more attractive
to the opposite sex............. 0 1 2 3

When things are going well for me, I feel less
dissatisfied with my body ... 0 1 2 3

(Adapted from "Taking Charge of Your Weight and Wellbeing" by Dr. Joyce Nash)

What your score means: If you scored under 15, you are fortunate in having a good body image and a high level of self-confidence. A score of 16 to 30 indicates a moderate dissatisfaction with your body and definite scope for improvement. If you scored more than 30, your body image is poor and you should take active steps to improve it. Pay attention to the steps outlined in this week's Behaviour section. Learn to judge yourself less harshly, to use criteria other than thinness by which to judge yourself and others, and to get support from a wider network of friends and activities. Join a group that examines issues related to body image or consider setting one up yourself. For information on courses, send a stamped addressed envelope to The Women's Therapy Centre, 6 Manor Gardens, London N7. For guidance on self-help therapy, read *In Our Own Hands* by Sheila Ernst and Lucy Goodison (Women's Press). There are fewer facilities available for men with these difficulties, but much of the information in the above book is applicable.

C FOR CONSUMPTION

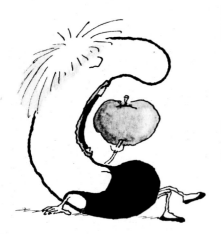

Before going on, review the progress you have made in the last two weeks. Check these points:

- Are you following the 10 recommendations made in Week One (eating wholemeal bread, cutting out sweets, chocolates, crisps etc)? Take another look at the list to jog your memory.
- Are you eating two apples a day?
- Have you given up sugar and reduced the amount of artificial sweetener you use? Try to give up artificial sweeteners now if you have not already, because, more than anything, sweet drinks help to maintain a taste for sweet food.
- Have you reduced your intake of alcohol, especially beer?

If you feel you want to follow a more demanding diet so as to slim more quicky, take these additional measures:

- Cut out roast or fried potatoes and chips.
- Substitute brown rice for white.
- Use meat as a flavouring or combined with other ingredients, not as a mainstay.

Eat it in stews, in pasta sauces, or mixed with beans.
- Eat four apples a day rather than feel hungry.

If you're not making as much progress as you would like because you are eating out often, use the following suggestions on what to order, whether in a smart restaurant or the local Chinese.

Eating Out

Cheaper restaurants

Italian or Chinese restaurants tend to be the best places for the high-carbohydrate style of eating recommended by the ABC Diet, though even there certain dishes can be traps for the unwary. Calorie values, where given in the guide that follows, are for comparison only.

Italian: Pasta is the obvious choice. Spaghetti Bolognese, which has a satisfying meat sauce, has only about 500 calories. With a Napoletana (tomato) sauce, there are even fewer.

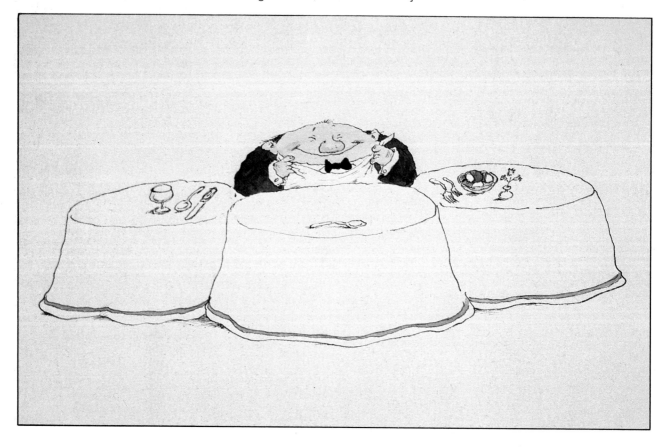

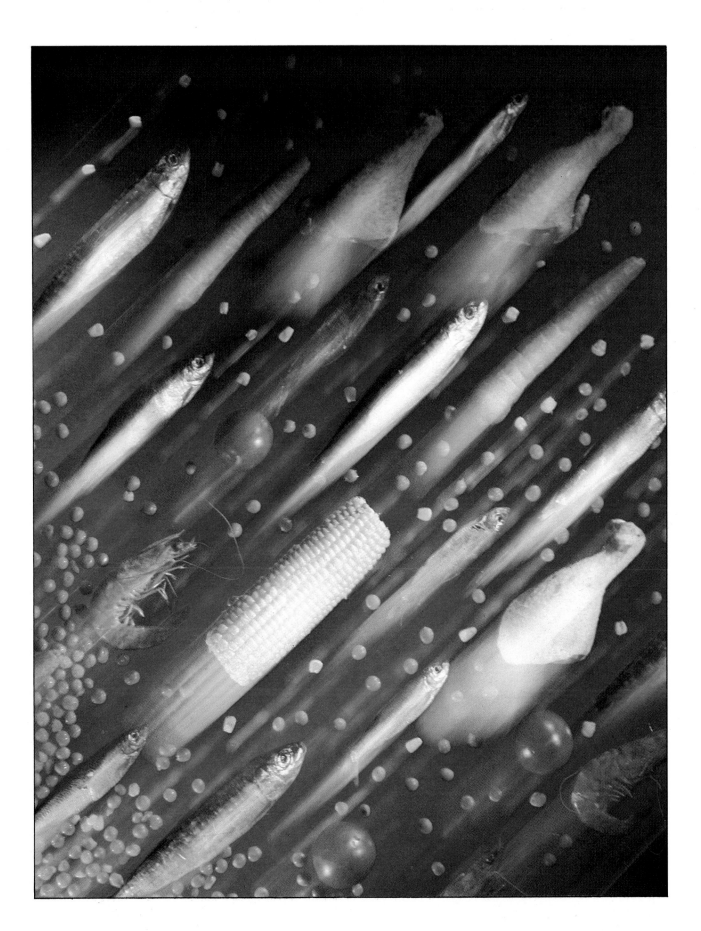

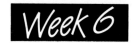

CONSUMPTION

Chinese: Choose dishes with plenty of beansprouts – they're filling, nutritious and low in calories. Chicken Chow Mein or Prawn Chop Suey with rice both have under 650 calories. Stay away from Sweet and Sour Pork: because of the deep fried batter and thick sweet sauce, a portion with rice comes to a disastrous 1150 calories. Egg Fu Yung is not much better.

Indian: Go for the tandoori dishes, which have no fat-laden sauce. Eat plain rice rather than fried, and chapati, nan or roti breads rather than the greasy parathas or puris. Raita (yoghurt with cucumber) is a good accompaniment.

Greek: One or two sticks of lamb or beef kebab with salad is a good choice. For a starter ask for tsatsiki (yoghurt with mint and cucumber) or a Greek salad with fetta cheese. Taramasalata is too oily. A little hummus (made from chick peas) would be better.

Fast foods and takeaways

Pizzas: Sizes vary, but an average fairly plain pizza, such a Napoletana or Veneziana, has about 600 calories. As a rule of thumb, the lower the price, the less cheese and the fewer calories you will get.

Baked potatoes: A very good choice, but be certain to ask for just a little butter. If you have a cheese, tuna or chilli filling – all fairly high in fat – skip the butter altogether.

Hamburgers: If you must, order the plain hamburger or cheeseburger. The chips, being thinly cut, are very high in fat – over 200 calories for a small portion at McDonald's, where the plain hamburger with bun has 260 calories and the cheeseburger an extra 45. At Wimpy a small cheeseburger or baconburger has about 350 calories. Don't be tempted by milk shakes, ice-cream floats, or apple pie, which range from 250 to 350 calories.

Fried chicken: Wimpy's chicken piece with chips has nearly 500 calories. A better choice, at around 400, is the chicken breast sandwich from Kentucky Fried Chicken.

Kebabs: The average doner kebab and salad in pitta bread amounts to about 550 calories and is one of the more satisfying fast food meals.

Fish and chips: Not for every day. The average helping has 770 calories, though you could save a bit by sharing a bag of chips and removing some of the batter.

Eating out in style

Going out to a good restaurant is many a slimmer's downfall. But a bit of care can keep you on the right tracks without making you feel left out.

The guidelines to follow are all common sense but worth repeating none the less. Drinks should be kept low in calories (see the table in Week One), rationed to two at most and supplemented with mineral or ordinary water. When it comes to food, the obvious trap to avoid is butter. Butter on bread, butter on vegetables, meat and fish drenched in butter – the fancier the establishment, the more they seem to use.

If you're likely to dull your appetite, not to say your outline, by eating half a dozen pieces of French bread and butter before the starter arrives, ask for it to be removed rather than twitch at the temptation. Ask for vegetables and salad to be served plain with butter or dressing on the side. The same goes for grilled fish or meat.

Clear soup, melon, perhaps with prosciutto, tomato juice or crudités without the aïoli, make good starters. Keep away from avocado, pâté or prawn cocktail. Avoid fried dishes; go instead for grilled or poached dishes, white fish and chicken especially. Game, being naturally low in fat, is a good choice so long as lots of fat hasn't been added in cooking. Choose vegetable-based sauces such as tomato, rather than creamy ones based on flour and butter. If you're eating pasta, have it Bolognese or Napoletana rather than al burro (with butter). Don't hesitate to ask how food is cooked.

There are few desserts that are not either too rich or too sugary to be advisable. Have a fruit salad if you wish, but plain fresh fruit is better. If you want cheese, go for Camembert or Brie (88 calories

per ounce) rather than Gorgonzola (112), Cheddar or Stilton (135). (Needless to say, leave out the butter.) Or skip the last course altogether and have coffee instead.

Quick Recipes for Slow Food

Prepared foods, from pork pies to TV dinners, are one of the slimmer's greatest hazards because they tend to be loaded with fat. To be certain that you are eating the right kind of food, you have to start with real ingredients, and that can take longer – although it need not. This week we explore two ways of producing 'slow' food fast – with the help of the freezer and the pressure cooker to save on shopping and cooking time. A well stocked freezer can give you vegetables almost as good as fresh – at least from the nutritional point of view – and a pressure cooker makes cheap and nourishing bean dishes more practical for the busy cook.

Lentil Soup

1 tbsp sunflower or olive oil; 4 rashers of back bacon, without rind and cut in pieces; 1 onion, chopped; 2 large carrots, sliced; 4 sticks celery, sliced; 8oz (225g) lentils, green or brown, picked over and washed; 1 bay leaf; 2 pints (1.2 litres) stock; salt and pepper; chopped parsley.

Heat the oil in the pressure cooker and fry the bacon. Add the vegetables to the pan, and cook over a medium heat until the onions are transparent. Then add the lentils, stock and bay leaf. Do not add salt at this stage. Bring to the boil, put on the lid, and let the pressure rise until it is hissing gently from under the weight. Cook for 5 minutes at high pressure (15lb/7kg) then allow the pressure to reduce slowly. Remove the bay leaf and adjust the seasoning. Either serve it as it is or put it through a Mouli-Légume or a food processor. Sprinkle with chopped parsley. This is a very filling soup and would make a good meal served with bread and cheese and a green salad.

Rice Pudding

2oz (50g) pudding rice; 1 pint (600ml) milk; 1oz (25g) unsalted butter; 1 egg, beaten with 1 tsp brown sugar; pinch of nutmeg or cinnamon; 1 bay leaf; 1 in (2.5cm) piece of lemon peel.

Melt the butter in the pressure cooker, add the milk, nutmeg or cinnamon, lemon peel and bay leaf. Bring to the boil, stir in the rice and adjust the heat so that the milk is simmering, not boiling up in the pan. Put on the lid and bring to high pressure (15lb/7kg). Cook for 12 minutes and allow the pressure to reduce slowly. Pour the pudding into a greased pie dish, stir in the egg beaten with the sugar and put it under a hot grill for a few minutes to brown the top.

It is also possible to bake this pudding in a low oven, 275°F (140°C, gas mark 1), for 2 hours. Cover the dish with a piece of oiled greaseproof paper and stir from time to time. Add the egg and sugar 10 minutes before the end of the cooking time and take the paper off to allow a skin to form.

Gammon with Baked Beans

1 small gammon joint (knuckle) or 4 slices of gammon; 12oz (350g) dried haricot or brown beans; 1 tbsp sunflower or olive oil; 1 onion, sliced; 6 tomatoes, cut in pieces, or one 15oz (425g) tin of tomatoes; 6 allspice berries; 2 tbsp black treacle; 1 tsp English mustard powder; 1½ pints (900ml) water; salt and pepper.

If you have a joint of gammon, soak it in cold water for 3 or 4 hours. Boil the beans in 3 pints of water for 1 minute, then leave to soak for 40 minutes. When you are ready to start cooking, put the gammon joint into a pan of fresh water and bring to the boil, remove it and put it on one side. There is no need to do this if you have gammon slices.

Heat the oil gently in the pressure cooker, add the onions, and fry them until they are transparent. Add the drained and rinsed beans, the tomatoes and the allspice berries. Mix the treacle and the mustard powder with a little hot water and pour over the beans. Put in the gammon and add the rest of the water. Bring to the boil, skim and adjust the heat so that the water is just boiling. Put on the lid and let the pressure build up. Time the cooking from the moment when the steam begins to escape from the weight. Cook at high pressure (15lb/7kg) for 35 minutes then reduce the pressure slowly. If the beans aren't quite cooked or there is too much liquid in the pan simmer with the lid off while you remove the gammon, take off the rind and any fat and discard the bones. Chop the meat and return to the pan. Add any seasoning necessary at this point.

It is also possible to cook the beans in a casserole. Bake in the oven at 300°F (150°C, gas mark 2) for 2½-3 hours, until the beans are soft and the gammon is cooked.

Trout Baked with Oats

4 frozen trout; 1½oz (40g) porridge oats; 1½oz (40g) chopped almonds; 2oz (50g) melted butter; salt and pepper

Take the trout from their wrapping. Mix the oatmeal with the chopped nuts and seasoning, put the mixture on a flat plate. Paint one side of each trout with melted butter, and press the buttered side of the fish down on to the oatmeal and nuts. Lay the fish on a greased fireproof dish with the oatmeal side underneath. Paint the top of the fish with butter and carefully press the rest of the oatmeal on to the surface of the fish. Trickle over any remaining butter, and bake in a preheated oven 400°F (200°C, gas mark 6), for 30 minutes.

Serve the fish with quarters of lemon, a crisp French loaf and a dish of green peas.

Vegetable Curry

1lb (450g) frozen cauliflower florets; 1lb (450g) other frozen vegetables: runner or French beans, sweetcorn, broccoli; 1 onion, chopped; 2 tbsp sunflower oil; 1 clove of garlic, crushed; 2 tbsp mild curry powder; 2oz (50g) dried coconut; 1 tbsp plain flour; 5oz (150g) yoghurt; salt and pepper; fresh coriander, or parsley, chopped; toasted almonds; salt and pepper.

Cook the vegetables except the onion separately (in boiling water): don't overcook them but keep them on the crisp side. Reserve a cupful of the cooking liquid for the sauce. Cover the vegetables with foil and put in a low oven while you make the sauce.

As the vegetables are cooking put the coconut in a measuring jug and fill it with ½ pint (300ml) of boiling water. Leave this to stand for 10 minutes. Fry the onion gently in the oil until soft. Add the garlic and curry powder and stir together, increasing the heat slightly. Add the flour, stir again and cook until thickened. Remove from the heat and stir in the strained coconut liquid a little at a time, return to the heat and cook a little longer. Stir in the yoghurt, add a few tablespoons of the vegetable water if necessary to make the sauce a nice consistency, like that of thick cream. Season the sauce, pour it over the vegetables, and decorate the top with toasted almonds and chopped fresh coriander or parsley. Serve with boiled rice and poppadums heated under the grill until crisp.

YOUR ABC DIARY: Week Five							Starting date:	
	WALKING		JOGGING/ WALKING		SWIMMING		HOME WORKOUT	OTHER EXERCISE (e.g. cycling)
	Mins	Miles*	Mins	Miles*	Mins	Lengths	Mins	Mins
Monday								
Tuesday								
Wednesday								
Thursday								
Friday								
Saturday								
Sunday								
TOTAL								

* approximate distance, optional

ABC ROAD TEST	mins		mph	SWIMMING TIME TEST		lengths	mins

BODY MEASUREMENTS	Date / /	Chest	Waist	Hips	Arms	Legs	Weight

WEEK 7

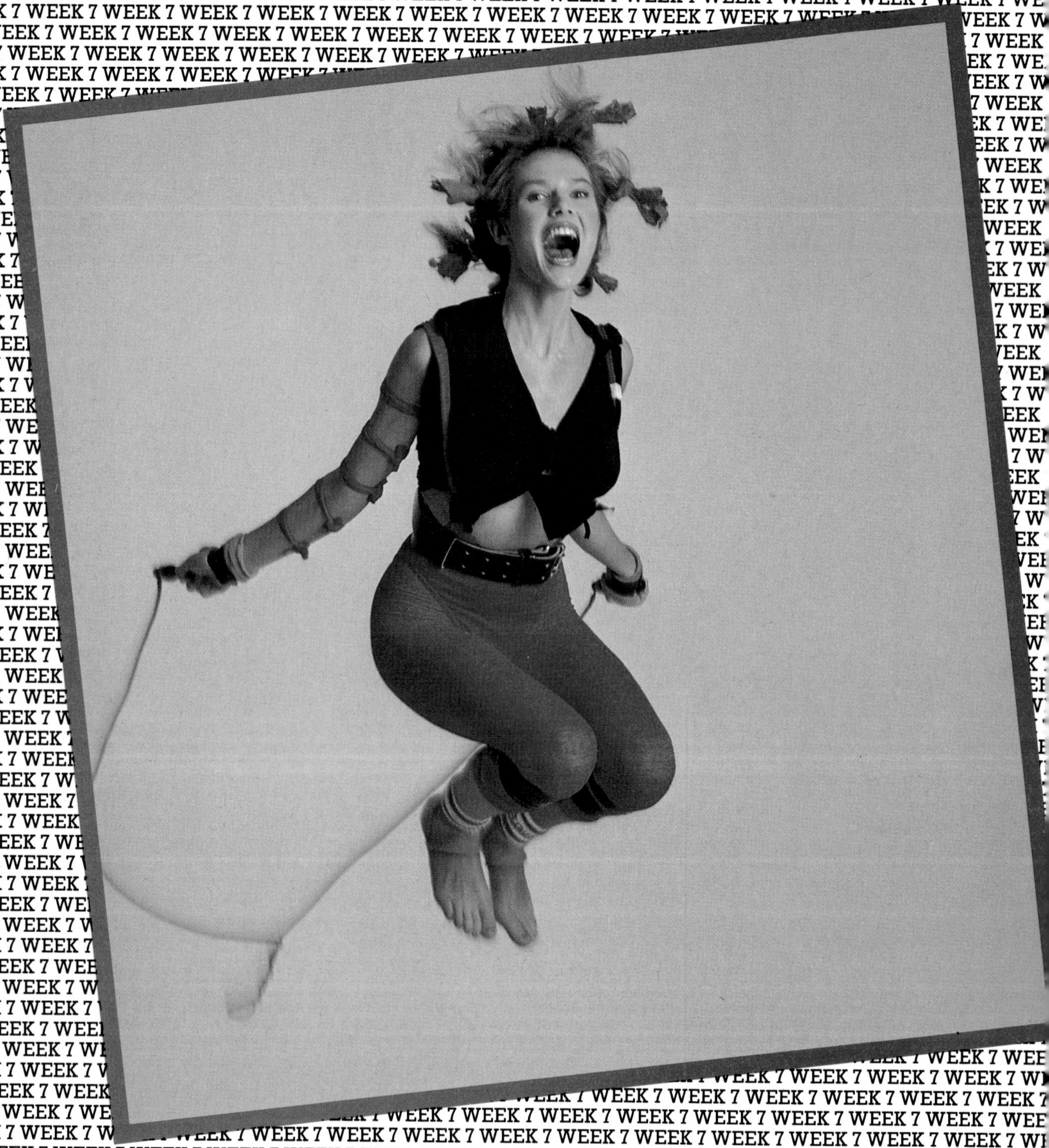

Week 7

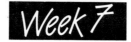

A FOR ACTIVITY

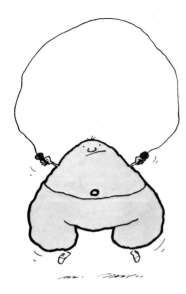

You have built up basic fitness – and can notice the rewards of your effort in a trimmer figure and a better feeling about yourself – now you can push yourself harder. Reach out for faster times, whether you are walking, running or swimming. If you are doing the Home Workout, demand more of yourself and experiment with new routines to add variety.

Do at least four exercise sessions this week (except for Walking Programme – see below).

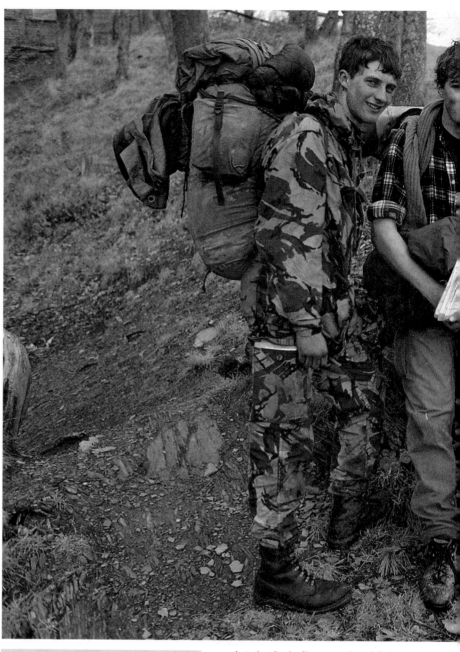

Walking Programme

Walk briskly for 30 to 40 minutes or more at least five times this week.

Dr Kenneth Cooper, who coined the word aerobics and has been largely responsible for popularizing aerobic exercising, has established norms of fitness, which are set out in his book *The New Aerobics.* A person of good to excellent fitness, in order to maintain their fitness, should, he says, walk

- three miles, five times a week, taking between 36 and 43 minutes, or
- four miles, five times a week, taking between 58 and 78 minutes, or
- four miles, three times a week, taking between 48 and 58 minutes.

These norms are for fitness. If you are already walking this far at this speed you have probably already become noticeably thinner. But if you have more fat to

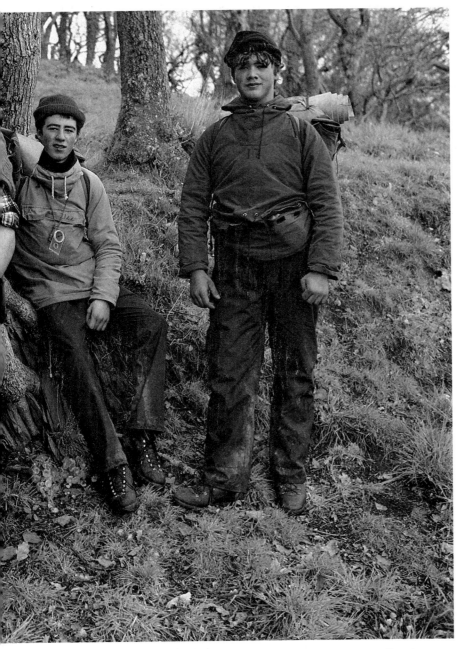

WALKING PLAN

stage	distance miles	time mins	times/ week	speed mph
1	1.5	30	6	3
2	2.0	40	5	3
3	2.0	40	6	3
4	2.0	36	5	3.3
5	2.0	36	6	3.3
6	2.0	33	5	3.6
7	2.0	33	6	3.6
8	2.5	42	5	3.6
9	2.5	42	6	3.6
10	2.5	39:30	5	3.8
11	2.5	39:30	6	3.8
12	2.5	37:30	5	4
13	2.5	37:30	6	4

You have now passed the ABC Road Test so you can do some gentle jogging if you want. Begin with no more than 20 to 30 seconds of gentle jogging two or three times during the walk. If you want to start jogging instead of walking then begin with Week One of our easy jogging programme.

14	3.0	45	5	4
15	3.0	45	6	4
16	3.0	43	5	4

You have now reached Dr Cooper's standard of aerobic fitness. Try to keep this up and reduce your time progressively for three miles towards 36 minutes (5 mph).

lose, you should walk six or seven times a week rather than the three to five times recommended by Cooper. If your progress has been slow because it has taken you time to reach a basic level of fitness – perhaps because you are very overweight – be reassured by the knowledge that once you are able to walk briskly your weight loss will be steady.

You may find it easier to make progress if you set definite goals as to time and distance. Whatever your level now, your ultimate goal should be to progress to one of Cooper's schedules outlined above. Use the walking plan set out in the panel to increase your speed gradually. Spend at least one week at each stage; accurately measure your route on a street map or ordnance survey map; determine from the last column the speed you should be aiming at in miles per hour; and record your progress in the ABC Diary. Do not be disheartened if your progress levels off for a time: this often happens in training. Persistence will pay off.

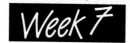

ACTIVITY

Jogging Programme

Jogging 1

Warm up with a brisk walk for five minutes.

Jog for five minutes, then walk for five minutes. Alternate jogging and walking for 35 minutes.

Finish with the Cool Down Stretches.

You can now attempt a three-mile course. Try to complete it in under 40 minutes (including the time spent walking to warm up), aiming to spend half the time jogging and the rest walking. Do it twice a week, or more if you can.

Jogging 2

Warm up for five minutes, walking briskly or jogging slowly.

Jog three miles or more, walking occasionally for five minutes if necessary.

Walk for a few minutes until you have cooled down.

Finish with the Cool Down Stretches.

Some days you may want to jog and walk four or five miles at a time; other days you may only feel like doing two. Running a longer distance once a week is a good way to vary your programme and gradually step up the demands you make on yourself. You might like to try, say, two three-mile jogs, a five-mile walk and jog, and a two-mile walk in the course of a week. The five-mile walk and jog will really stretch you, so choose the time carefully: the weekend may be best. You could then do the two-mile walk on the other weekend day, taking friends or family with you.

Swimming Programme

Swimming 1

Swim 20 lengths.

Do the Figure Trimming Exercises.

Twenty lengths of 25 metres each add up to 500 metres or almost a third of a mile. This is something like the length you need to swim regularly in order to get thinner. If you can manage 20 uninterrupted lengths, you can drop the Pool Exercises, doing them if you want to for variety. Continue with the Figure Trimming Exercises.

Swimming 2

Swim 34 lengths (850 metres or just over half a mile), changing strokes every two or three lengths and resting if you need to every eight or 10 lengths.

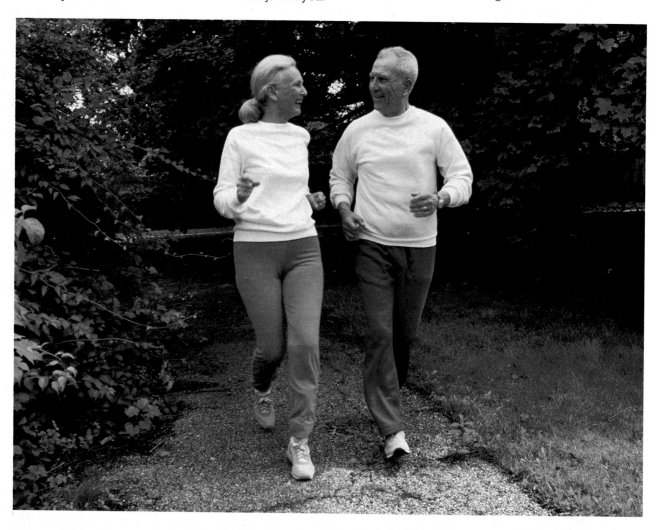

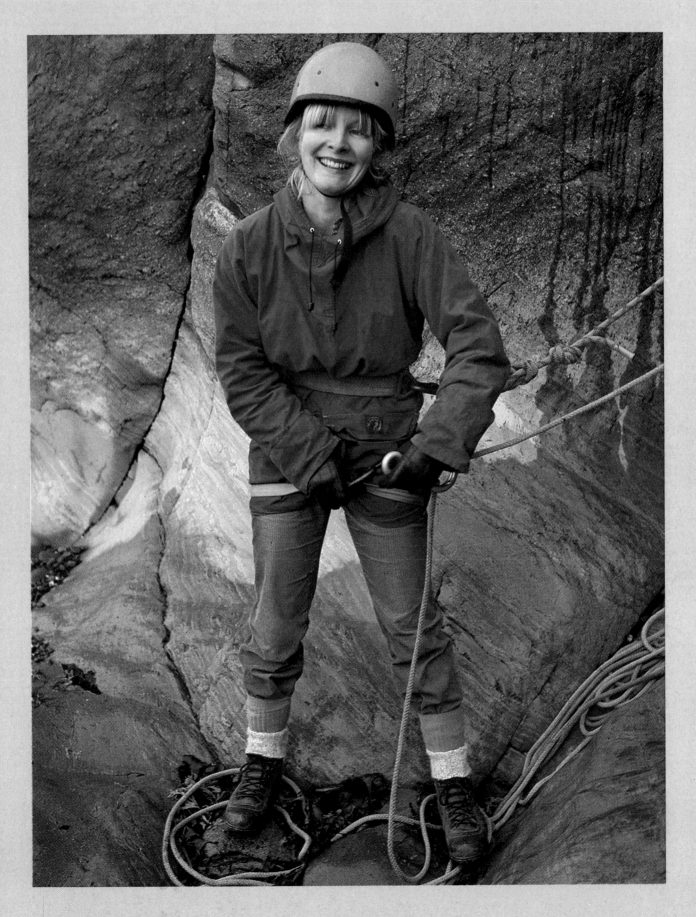

ACTIVITY

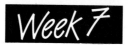

The Home Workout

If your routine is taking more than 40 minutes, cut out any section of the Home Workout that you find unappealing and make up the time with movement you enjoy, but keep it vigorous.

Here are two more advanced exercises to tighten the muscles of your abdomen. Follow the instructions carefully to avoid injury.

Bent Knee Curl-Ups. This exercise will help strengthen weak abdominal muscles. It should at no time be felt in the lower back. Lie on the floor with your knees bent, legs parallel and feet flat on the floor. Pull your abdominal muscles in hard so that you can feel the lower back being pressed down into the floor. Resting your hands flat on the outside of your thighs, tuck in your chin, then curl the top half of the body up off the floor. If the abdominal muscles are very weak from neglect you will not be able to curl up very far at first. Do not try to jerk yourself up, but keep the movement slow and smooth. Breathe out as you curl up, and in as you slowly lower yourself. If you feel the neck and shoulders becoming very tight, try resting a cushion under your head. Do this eight times slowly then 16 times quickly if you can. Bend your knees into your chest to release when you have finished.

Buttock Squeezes. Still lying down, place your feet flat on the floor, with your knees bent, and legs parallel. Pull in your abdominal muscles and tilt the pelvis upwards, then lift your buttocks off the floor without allowing your back to arch. Hold this position and make small pushing up movements, tightening the buttocks each time you push upwards. Do not allow your bottom to touch the floor between push-ups. Repeat until your muscles feel well worked (but not burning from muscle fatigue). Now bend your knees and squeeze them into your chest to release muscles. Then roll on to your side and stand up.

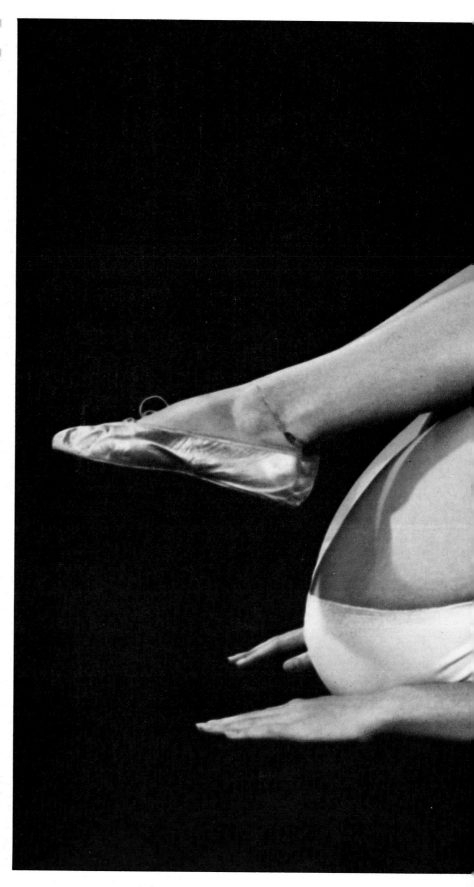

Marilyn Monroe works out, in 1949, aged 23.

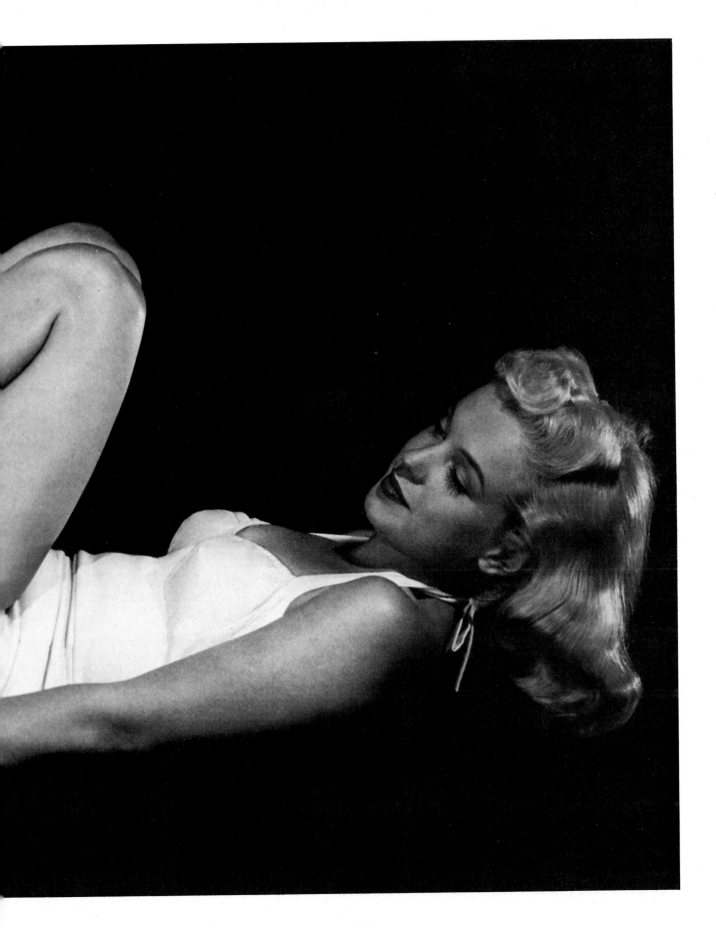

B FOR BEHAVIOUR

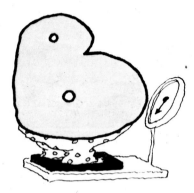

No one need be a victim of their biography, said the American psychologist George Kelly, meaning that as we make ourselves the way we are, we have the power to remake ourselves. In order to cast off old ways, however, we must realize that they actually serve a purpose in our lives which needs to be understood before they can be discarded. You may have been overweight all your adult life. This doesn't mean that you are doomed to remain overweight for ever. If you can find out and acknowledge what it is that's holding you back, you will be able to change for good, not just temporarily. What appears to be just a deplorable nuisance may be useful in the context of your life because of the meanings you have attached to it. Pinpointing those meanings will help you to stop sabotaging your own efforts.

Escape from History

This week's exercise explores the notion that you can find out if a problem has a deeper meaning for you. Based on the personal construct psychology (PCP) of the late George Kelly, professor of psychology at Boston's Brandeis University, it is fun to do, yet it is also remarkably powerful and can produce valuable information which would take a long time to arrive at by other methods. We suggest you do it with a good friend, who can write down your answers as they come up. Answers should be set out as in the examples given below.

1. **Define a problem you would like to explore related to your weight.** The greater the emotional charge of the problem you pick, the more fruitful the exercise is likely to be. If you are someone who has been on many diets, only to gain back the inches lost, you can usefully take your size as a starting point. Define the problem as, say, 'fatness' or 'being fat', or, as in the example of Anne below, 'being fat and lumpy'. Do not worry too much about the exact words: this is a first step only. If you have had trouble sticking to one part of the ABC Bodyplan, you could define your problem as 'overeating', or 'not exercising enough', or 'drinking too much', depending on your particular difficulty. This is referred to as *the problem*.

2. **Without attempting to monitor or censor your thoughts, write down all the words or phrases that come into your mind in connection with the problem.** Do not spend more than five minutes on this, and don't think about it too hard. The answers should be spontaneous. From this list, pick a word or phrase that you consider represents an important aspect of the problem. This is referred to as *the symptom*.

3. **Find the opposite of the symptom.** It need not be the dictionary opposite. This is the desired alternative to the symptom and is known as *the jackpot*.

4. **List the disadvantages of the symptom.** This is *the handicap*.
5. **List the advantages of the jackpot.** These are called *the winnings*.
6. **List the advantages of the symptom.** This is *the payoff*.
7. **List the disadvantages of the jackpot.** This is *the cost*.

This exercise does not entail delving around in your past to find the reasons for your problem or stirring up the unconscious in search of motives. However, it is very informative, in spite of its relative simplicity. It assumes that any habitual problem – the symptom – also has its positive aspects – the payoff. The payoff is probably much less obvious, especially to the person who seems to be running around in circles. The jackpot (the desired alternative to the symptom) also has both positive and negative implications – these are the winnings and the cost, respectively.

Seen in this light, every problem, and every symptom of that problem, is in effect a dilemma: when you try to discard the symptom so as to reach the jackpot, you are faced with the cost, the price to be paid for achieving your objective.

You must first decide if the cost is too high. If it is, you can start looking for ways of achieving the jackpot without losing the payoff, or of enjoying the payoff without having to suffer the symptom.

In examining your responses, it may seem to you that you cannot combine the winnings with the payoff. At this point, you need to look for alternative ways of viewing the problem. Look again at the jackpot and items listed in the winnings category and ask yourself if they belong together, if they really are desirable, and if new ways can be found to reach them. Tackling a problem head on can arouse anxiety if alternative means are not found of enjoying the advantages it confers. The motto is: ignore the payoff at your peril.

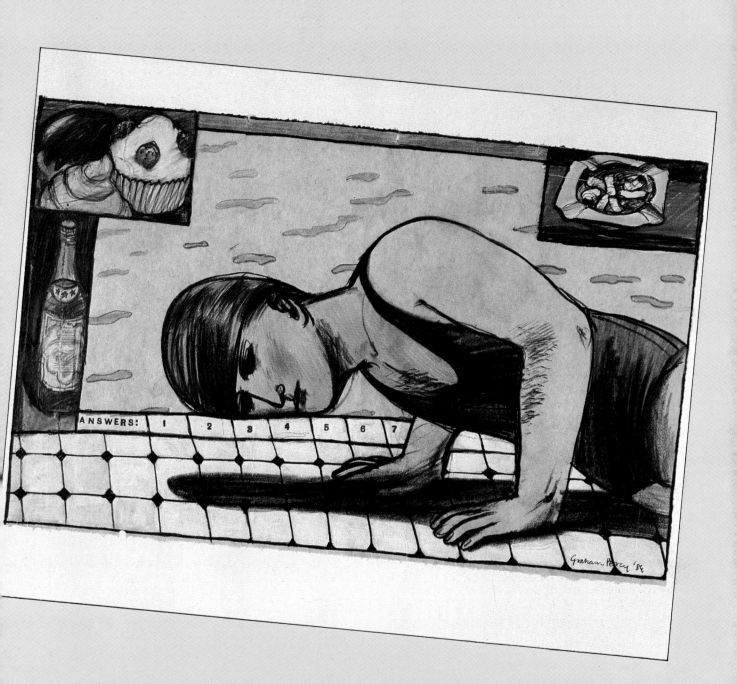

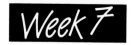

BEHAVIOUR

Anne's dilemma

Here is an example to illustrate the PCP exercise: Anne is 33, single, and works for a multinational company, making all the travel and removal arrangements for executives going abroad. She lives alone. Anne defines her problem as 'being big and lumpy'. From the list of words and phrases that free association produces, she picks the word 'unpopular' as a key symptom. The opposite for her – the jackpot – is 'to be sought after' Her answers can be tabulated as follows:

1. *The problem*. Being big and lumpy.
2. *The symptom*. Unpopular.
3. *The jackpot* (opposite of the symptom). To be sought after.
4. *The handicap* (disadvantages of being unpopular). Spend too much time at home. Feel sorry for myself. Don't think highly of my boyfriends.
5. *The winnings* (advantages of being sought after). Would have more fun. Wouldn't need to pretend to be happy. More attention from men. More respect at work.
6. *The payoff* (advantages of being unpopular). More time to be creative. Don't arouse envy and hostility. Avoid leading shallow existence.
7. *The cost* (disadvantages of being sought after). No time to myself. Others envious.

Anne's dilemma lies in wanting to be sought after without arousing envy and without being left with too little time to be creative and caring. She needs to find ways of being creative and of helping others without making herself unpopular – in other words, she has to find a way to make creativity and helpfulness compatible in her view of things with social and professional success, fun and happiness. Then she will get both the jackpot and the winnings.

It seems Anne is attributing to slimness an almost magical quality it does not necessarily possess. In her mind, slimness confers not only popularity (the jackpot) but fun, happiness, attention from men and respect at work (the winnings). If she does become slim, she will quite probably be disappointed, for her expectations are not realistic. While slimness may certainly bring more attention from men (indeed this is why some women stay fat) there is no guarantee of automatic happiness or respect at work, both of which have to be earned. Anne should ask herself if she is blaming her weight for an unsatisfactory life instead of taking steps to make her life more fulfilling through friendships, work, hobbies and recreation.

Other issues are raised by her answers. Being sought after does not rule out being creative nor does it necessarily mean being left with no time to oneself. Anne needs to consider whether she finds it a problem to refuse the demands of others and is using her size as a way of saying 'no'. She should also look at how she will respond to any increased sexual demands she may encounter if she loses weight. She further needs to consider why she brackets social popularity with selfishness and whether she has created a false equation. Why should being popular entail leading a 'shallow existence'?

Also worth considering is why she has a poor opinion of her boyfriends. It is possible that she has a poor opinion of herself and does not feel she deserves relationships with men she respects, or perhaps she undervalues her boyfriends simply because they show an interest in her. (Many fat women find it hard to believe that the men in their life like them the way they are.) She should look for ways of increasing her self-esteem that do not revolve around size or weight. Lastly, Anne lists one of the payoffs of being unpopular as not arousing envy and hostility. Is she prepared to brave a certain amount of possible envy and hostility as the price of slimness? If not, she is likely to put weight on again as a retreat to safety. In answering these questions Anne will identify some of the psychological influences which are preventing her from losing weight permanently.

For more information about personal construct psychology, and the special groups for slimmers using this approach, contact the Centre for Personal Construct Psychology, 132 Warwick Way, London SW1.

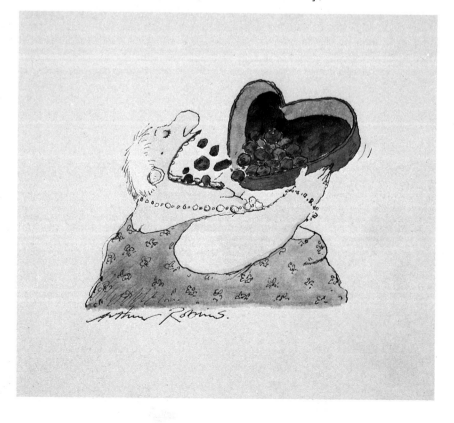

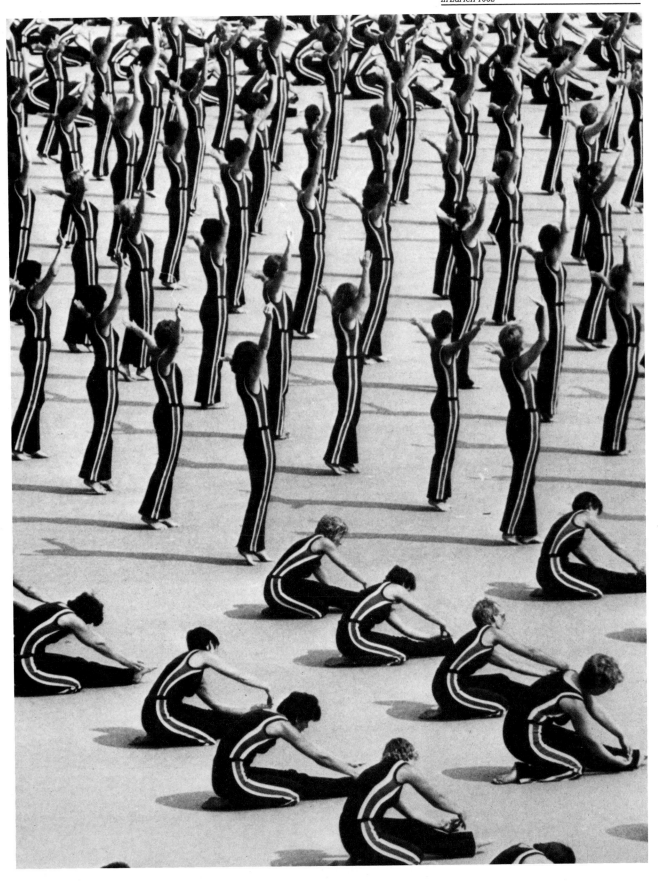

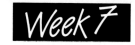

C FOR CONSUMPTION

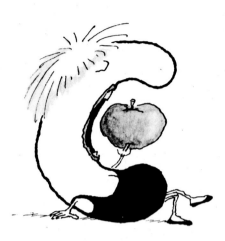

If you are still not improving in shape or losing weight fast enough, and you have followed our dietary recommendations, it could be that you are eating too much and need to take more direct control of your food consumption. We don't think it is a good idea to restrict your intake by counting calories because it is one of the least popular ways of slimming. A MORI poll for the Sunday Times *has found that slimmers much prefer cutting down on food to counting calories (see panel in Week One). In any case most calorie-controlled diets encourage you to starve yourself rather than to try to achieve a natural control of appetite.*

Speeding up Your Weight Loss

So we suggest another approach to restricting your food consumption, one which develops natural appetite control. It should appeal to people who have regular eating habits but are not improving in shape as fast as they would like. It should also prove helpful to people who, because of their age or ill health, find they can only progress slowly with the exercise plan. However, it is vital to keep going with exercise and to review the suggestions we have made about dietary changes and eating behaviour. If snacking or bingeing is your problem, then this approach will not help.

Sizing up the cake

This method of controlling food consumption is based on the simple fact that most people find it easy to judge whether a slice of cake, or any portion of food, is bigger or smaller than a helping of the same food eaten a day or two previously. Most people find this easy although they would find it difficult, if not impossible, to judge the number of calories in the same items.

The key is to eat just a little less at each meal than you have in the past. Do not attempt to make any dramatic reductions in your food intake. You should never feel really hungry or dissatisfied after a meal – if you do you are cutting down too much. Just try to cut out a little of each food you eat. You need only make a small reduction in food intake to lose weight in the long run.

This is how to do it:
1. *Reduce helpings.* Cut down on the amount you usually eat but avoid cutting out any particular food such as potatoes or bread, since this would make your meal unbalanced. If the meal is served to you, then you may have to leave just a little of everything on the plate. This means overcoming feelings of guilt about leaving food.
2. *Cut out starters or dessert.* This can also be an effective strategy but you may find it makes you feel deprived – and what do you do while everyone else is eating? In the long term it is more sensible to ask for a small helping, or to accept a normal helping and leave some of it. Learning to leave food on your plate is a valuable habit to acquire.
3. *Be selective about what you leave on your plate,* especially avoiding items that are high in sugar and/or fat. Use the guidelines on cutting empty calories in the 10 rules for a better diet given in Week One.
4. *Don't be tempted to skip meals,* because of the danger that it may lead to a starve-and-stuff routine. If you know you won't have time for a proper meal break, take sandwiches and/or fruit with you.

WHY CALORIES DON'T COUNT

The number of calories a person needs or uses up during an average day varies greatly depending on their size, their age, and the amount of exercise they take. An "average" person might use 2,500 calories a day and eat approximately the equivalent in food, whereas an athlete might use up and eat almost twice as much. The amount of ordinary everyday activity engaged in makes a great difference to the amount of food needed to fuel the body. This is shown by the story of 1,154 Irish brothers who have been studied in a major research project. If you never thought you would be able to have your cake and eat it, this shows you how you can.

The Irish brothers were chosen in pairs – one brother lived in Boston, Massachusetts, and the other brother lived in Ireland. The brothers living in Ireland consumed 3,768 calories a day on average – 700 calories more than their Boston brothers. Yet the brothers living in Ireland who were eating more weighed on average 10 pounds less. The Irish brothers were physically more active than their Boston brothers and so they could eat more and weigh less.

This difference of 700 calories between the consumption of the brothers in Boston and Ireland is equivalent to an average serving of fish and chips, three pints of beer, four ounces of sweets and a Mars bar, or a dozen biscuits. So the lesson of the Irish brothers is that you can eat more if you take exercise and yet actually weigh less.

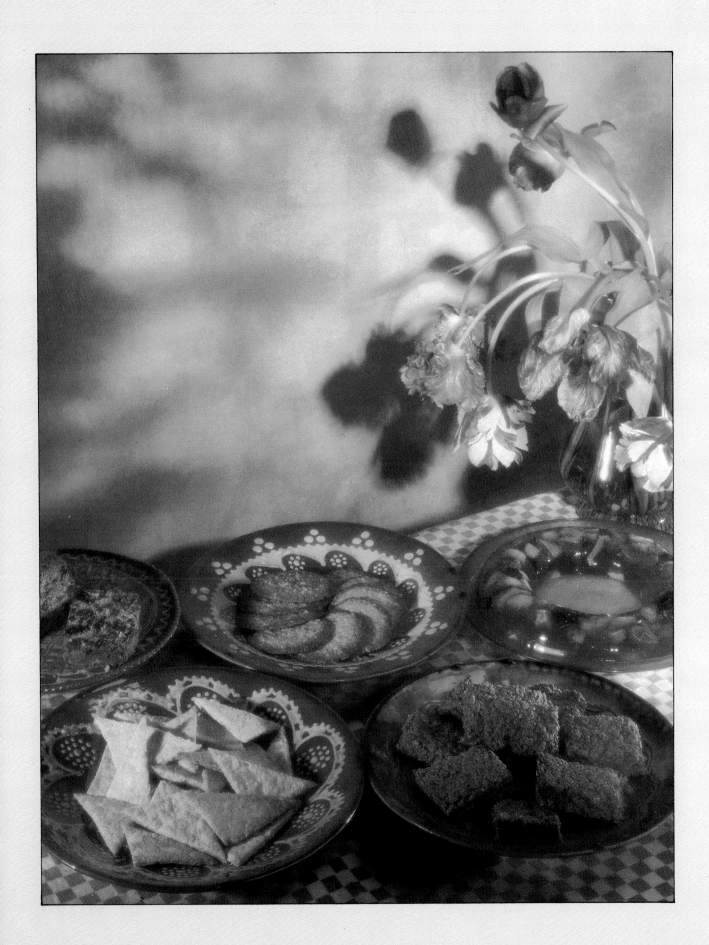

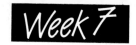

CONSUMPTION

High Tea

Some slimmers fear the English tea as the meal they are most likely to regret. But that need not be the case.

If you find it difficult to believe that it is possible to slim by eating bread, the teatime staple, then listen to this advice from Dr Olaf Mickelson, professor of nutrition at Michigan University: 'Bread in large amounts is an ideal food in a weight reducing regime. Recent work in our laboratory indicates that slightly overweight young men lost weight in a painless and practically effortless manner when they included 12 slices of bread per day in their programme. That bread was eaten with their meals. As a result, they became satisfied before they consumed their usual quota of calories. The subjects were admonished to restrict those foods that were concentrated sources of energy (ie. high in calories); otherwise, they were free to eat as much as they desired'. Over a period of eight weeks eight men lost an average of over 19 pounds in weight on this diet, eating high-fibre bread. Another group of eight men who ate bread which looked the same but was lower in fibre lost only 14 pounds.

Our high tea recipes have been created to reduce the excess sugar and fat which cause problems for slimmers and to provide a meal balanced to give lasting energy together with plenty of fibre and nutrients.

Recipes

Fruit Cake

4oz (100-125g) butter; 2oz (50g) sugar, golden granulated or light brown; 4oz (100-125g) self-raising flour; 1 tsp mixed spice; pinch salt; 12oz (350g) dried fruit such as apricots, peaches, prunes, pears, figs, apple; 2 fl oz (50m) milk, approximately; 1 egg, beaten.

Cream the butter and sugar until light and fluffy. Sift the flour with the spices and a pinch of salt. Cut up the fruit into small pieces, using a spoonful of the flour to coat the pieces and make them easier to cut. Mix the flour and the fruit into the creamed butter and sugar, adding enough milk to make a stiff mixture. Stir in the well-whisked egg. Line an 8x4 (20x10cm) loaf tin

with greased foil or butter paper and fill it with the mixture, levelling the top. Tie a double layer of brown paper round the outside of the tin. Cook in a low oven, 275°F (140°C, gas mark 1) for 2½ to 3 hours, testing with a skewer to see if the cake is done.

Flapjacks

Makes 12 – 16

4oz (100-125g) apple and pear spread*; 2 tbsps golden syrup; 4oz (100-125g) butter; 8oz (225g) porridge, Scott's or Quaker oats; salt; 1 tsp ginger.

Pre-heat oven to 350°F (180°C, gas mark 4). Melt the apple and pear spread with the golden syrup and the butter until liquid, not too hot. Beat well and add to the oats, salt and ginger, mixing all together. Pack firmly into a lined and greased 7 inch (17.5cm) square tin and level the top of the mixture with a spatula. Cook for 20-25 minutes until golden brown. Cut the flapjack into 12-16 pieces and leave to cool in the tin.

* This is made from fruit alone, with no added sugar, and can replace some of the sugar in cakes and biscuits. There are two brands available in health stores, at about £1 for 1 lb: Sunwheel Foods Ltd (Granary Health, Welmore Road, Burton-on-Trent, Staffs) and Whole Earth (Unit D, Western Trading Estate, Park Royal Road, London NW10).

Orange Oat Cookies

Makes 18-20

3oz (75g) butter; 2oz (50g) sugar, golden granulated or soft brown; 1 orange, grated rind and 3 tbsp juice; 2oz (50g) plain flour, sifted; 1oz (25g) ground almonds; 1oz (25g) porridge oats; pinch salt

Cream the butter and sugar, gradually adding the orange juice. Mix in the orange rind, flour, ground almonds, oats and salt. Put teaspoons of the mixture on to a greased baking sheet, leaving room for the cookies to spread. Bake in a 350°F (180°C, gas mark 4) oven for 10-12 minutes. Cool on a baking rack.

Oat Biscuits to Serve with Cheese

1½oz (30g) butter; 3oz (75g) porridge, Scott's or Quaker oats; 3oz (75g) plain flour; ½ tsp baking powder; pinch salt; 3 fl oz (75ml) boiling water

Rub the butter into the oats, flour, salt and baking powder. Pour on a little boiling water to make a stiff dough. Allow to cool then roll out on a floured board to the thickness of a 10p piece. Cut into rectangles or triangles or use a round cutter and arrange the biscuits on a greased baking sheet. Cook in a moderate oven, 350°F (180°C, gas mark 4) for 12 minutes. Remove from the oven and turn the biscuits over, cook for 5 more minutes or until the biscuits are a pale gold colour. Serve with cheese.

Apple Jelly

This is a sugar-free pudding with a spicy flavour; the addition of the dried fruit makes it more interesting than jelly by itself. Serve it with yoghurt or a mixture of yoghurt and cream. Start to make this the

day before you need it.

4oz (100-125g) dried fruit salad (apples, pears, apricots, figs and prunes) chopped and soaked; 1 pint (600ml) unsweetened apple juice; 3 or 4 cloves; 1 inch of cinnamon stick; rind of 1 lemon; 1 (0.4oz/11g) packet of gelatine; 2 fl oz (50ml) whipping cream; 3 or 4 tbsp yoghurt

Rinse the fruit and chop it into small pieces, removing the stones from the prunes. Leave it to soak in the apple juice overnight. The next morning strain a quarter of a pint (150ml) of the juice into a small pan and simmer gently for 10 minutes with the spices and the pared rind of the lemon. Strain this hot juice and return it to the pan away from the heat. Allow to cool a moment or two. Sprinkle in the gelatine and stir to dissolve. Remove the fruit from the juice and arrange it in a jelly mould, either a plain one or a ring mould. Mix the juice with the gelatine and gradually ladle it into the mould so as not to disturb the fruit; don't worry if some apple floats to the surface. Put the jelly in a cold place to set. Turn out by dipping the mould into hot water while you count to 10. It will help to loosen round the edge of the mould with a thin knife first.

Beat the cream and gently mix in the yoghurt. Serve in a bowl with the jelly.

Chick Pea and Mushroom Pâté

3oz (75g) butter; 6oz (150g) cooked chick peas; 4oz (100-125g) button mushrooms, cleaned and chopped into ¼ inch pieces; 1 tbsp lemon juice; small bunch parsley; 1 tbsp tahini (a paste made with toasted sesame seeds, obtainable in health food shops and some ethnic stores); salt and pepper

Melt 2oz (50g) of the butter and blend with the chick peas, lemon juice, tahini, parsley, salt and pepper in a food processor or liquidizer. Melt the remaining butter in a non-stick frying pan and cook the cleaned and chopped mushrooms for 5 minutes until they are just beginning to brown a little. Increase the heat and evaporate any liquid in the pan. Check the seasoning of the pâté and stir in the mushroom pieces. (This can be done in the processor but it is really nicer to have the mushrooms in pieces.) Decorate with a little chopped parsley and serve with hot pitta bread as part of a high tea. It also makes a good snack, or can be served as a first course.

Kedgeree with Kippers

8oz (225g) long grain rice; 2 eggs; 3 or 4 kippers or 6 or 8 kipper fillets; 2oz (50g) butter; parsley; salt and pepper

Cook the rice with a little salt until just done. Meanwhile boil one of the eggs for 10 minutes, cool a little in cold water and peel. Cook the kippers and remove the flesh in pieces from the bones and skin. (The easiest method is to put the kippers in a tall jug and to pour enough boiling water over them to cover. Put a plate on top of the jug and leave for about 8 minutes.) When the rice is cooked, drain it and return to the pan, quickly add the butter, the chopped egg white and the kipper flakes. Check the seasoning. Beat the remaining egg and stir it in carefully to coat the rice and fish. Serve on a hot dish sprinkled with the chopped egg yolk and parsley. It is possible to substitute smoked haddock for kipper or to use freshly cooked salmon.

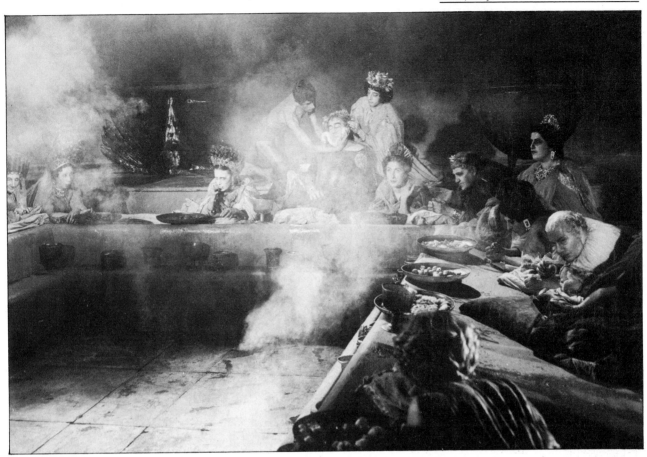

Trimalchio's feast, in Fellini's 'Satyricon' (United Artists, 1969).

YOUR ABC DIARY: Week Seven					Starting date:		
	WALKING		JOGGING/ WALKING		SWIMMING		HOME WORKOUT	OTHER EXERCISE (e.g. cycling)
	Mins	Miles*	Mins	Miles*	Mins	Lengths	Mins	Mins
Monday								
Tuesday								
Wednesday								
Thursday								
Friday								
Saturday								
Sunday								
TOTAL								

* approximate distance, optional

ABC ROAD TEST	mins		mph		SWIMMING TIME TEST	lengths	mins
BODY MEASUREMENTS	Date / /	Chest	Waist	Hips	Arms	Legs	Weight

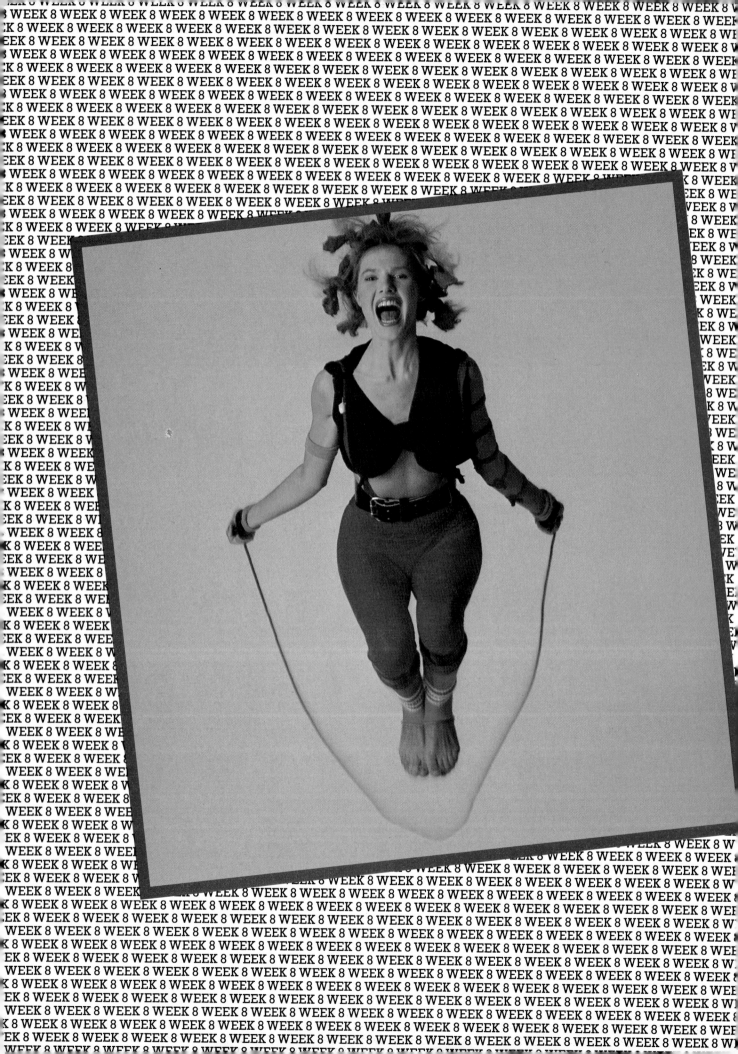

Week 8

A FOR ACTIVITY

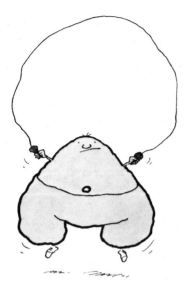

The ABC Bodyplan is intended to be a lifetime programme. We chose an eight week period to introduce it because that is just long enough to see some results for all your hard work. By now you should have gained some muscle and become addicted to exercise.

After eight weeks of exercise you are probably in the top 10 per cent of your age group for fitness – wherever you were at the beginning. You should now be able to run for a bus with ease, and when you have to work long hours for some reason, or have difficult days at home, you should have the extra stamina to see you through. You have also almost certainly lost weight. Even if you have only lost a little, you will certainly have become slimmer and a better shape.

If you want to slim still further, you should plan to keep exercising at least four times a week until you reach a stable weight. After that you may be able to cut down to three times a week, but that is the minimum for staying slim – unless you prefer to go back to starvation methods to control your weight. You may find it easier to keep up with your exercise if you have some outside goal to work towards, or if you join a group or sports club.

Do at least four exercise sessions this week (except for Walking Programme – see below).

Walking Programme

By now you may have walked 100 miles as part of this programme. You should be settling into a definite routine and have found easy ways of including walking in your day. Keep working on improving your time and distance, using the table we gave you last week, and keep doing the exercises to strengthen abdominal muscles.

To introduce more variety into your exercise programme, do the Home Workout or swim once or twice a week. If you want to start jogging, begin at Week One with the easy jogging programme.

Jogging Programme

Jogging 1

If you are jogging comfortably for five minutes at a time, see if you can extend your jog to eight or 10 minutes of uninterrupted running.
- After warming up, jog for eight to 10 minutes.
- Walk for a few minutes.
- Repeat jogging and walking sequence, then cool down, to make a total of 30 to 40 minutes.
- Finish with the Cool Down Stretches.

If by the end of this week you are doing jogs of eight to 10 minutes and you want to work up to continuous jogging, start next week on Week Four of Jogging 2. Work steadily through Jogging 2, taking more than a week over each stage if you need it.

Alternatively, if you are happy jogging for three to five minutes at a time with brisk walks in between, continue doing so. But lengthen outings to about 40 minutes so that you are covering a good distance. Continue to keep a record of progress.

Jogging 2

- You should now be able to jog continuously for about 30 to 40 minutes. In that time you should aim to cover three to four miles. If you can do five you are doing well. You can if you wish now begin your jog with a minute's walk, followed by rather slow jogging for a few minutes to warm up. You will soon learn to know when you feel fully warmed up and can increase your stride. Finish by walking about for a minute. Continue to keep an exercise diary so that you can monitor your progress. You will almost certainly get down to the size you want with four 40 minute jogs a week. If you then want to enhance your fitness for its own sake, start trying to improve your time.
- Always finish with the Cool Down Stretches.

Swimming Programme

Swimming 1

This plan was designed for people who started out less than fit. If you have kept up with the plan and can complete 20 lengths without undue difficulty or tiredness, you are now well above average fitness and can try your first time test.

Time test: Begin by swimming four lengths to warm up. Now swim non-stop for 15 minutes at a steady pace you think you can keep up without strain. Change strokes as you wish and try not to stop for a rest if you can help it. Record the number of lengths you swim in 15 minutes in the ABC Diary and check your pulse to see if it is within the training range for your age. Repeat this test regularly to assess your progress.

Swimming 1 and 2: How to continue the swimming programme

Your aim now should be to get at least half an hour of continuous exercise in the swimming pool four times a week. This does not mean you have to plough up and down doing length after length and nothing else. It is much better if you can split your time up a bit to add variety and interest.

Eventually your total swimming session should last 45 minutes. The time might be planned something like this:
1. 5 minutes' vigorous warm up – make use of the Pool Exercises.

2. 15 minutes swimming lengths, concentrating on correct breathing and on getting a strong pull through the water.
3. 5 minutes' Figure Trimming Exercises at the side of the pool.
4. 15 minutes swimming lengths, alternating strokes and using side or backstroke if you like these.
5. 5 minutes' fun.

Keep a check on the number of lengths you do and try to increase it in each 15 minute session. You should find the number slowly builds up. When you have an occasional off day you may want only a short swim. That doesn't matter. It is important to enjoy exercising so that you keep it up.

The Home Workout

If you are enjoying your Home Workout, keep going. To make a change, you could go back to the beginning of this book and start on the Jogging 1 or one of the swimming plans. If you can't swim you could have lessons. Age is no bar to learning to swim – plenty of people have learnt in their 60s or 70s. Whatever other exercise activities you take on, do the Home Workout on one or two of the four exercise sessions a week.

How to Continue to Keep Fit

Running

You don't have to train for a marathon to compete in running events at a recreational level. The great proof is The Sunday Times National Fun Run, the first national event of the recreational boom in Britain. Entries for this modest 2½ mile run have risen from 12,000 for the first Fun Run in 1978 to 29,000 in 1983. The popularity of the event stems from the fact that everyone runs in his or her own age group, from the under-10s to the over-60s, with many of those in the field running times which are well within the compass of the average person.

The Fun Run has encouraged many once-a-year groups to form clubs to explore the now lengthy programme of running events, including fun runs, half-marathons and established events on the club athletics calendar (see 'More information', note 1).

Fell running

Especially in the North, fell running provides a more strenuous version of athletics; but, while it may be more demanding at the sharp end, this sport also happily accommodates those of modest ability (2).

Orienteering

Most modest of all, perhaps, is orienteering, a sport which structures its competitions into many different age categories and degrees of expertise. It is a very accessible sport: a great many events can be entered on the day by complete beginners (3).

Ball games

Another growth sport is badminton, which, as well as proving popular with families, is thought to be one of the best sports for the elderly. Almost all sports centres have badminton courts and many have beginners' courses in badminton and squash.

Such courses are likely to provide a natural introduction to club competition. Indeed, the best way to look for a club for such sports is probably to ask your local sports centre.

Lawn tennis clubs are likely to be longer established and better known. They are also likely to welcome new members of modest ability; although you have to be 'played in' to be accepted, the standard is not high. A tennis club gives you plenty of competition at your own level, including the opportunity to take part in veterans' events at local and national level.

Cycling

Of the 'pure' exercise sports, cycling is a classic which, like athletics, is starting to accommodate a surge of newcomers. Cycling clubs have a strong tradition of veterans' racing, and there are also touring clubs (4).

Swimming

Swimming remains a disappointment among fitness sports. Pools are certainly beginning to cater for exercise swimming but, with swimming *clubs* apparently interested only in speedy youngsters, there is little opportunity for recreational swimmers to enjoy competition of the sort now available to runners.

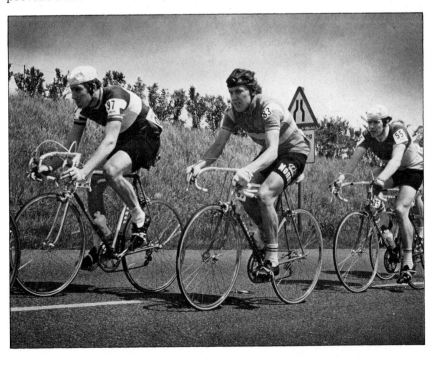

ACTIVITY

Triathlon

Ironically, the easiest way to engage in this type of swimming competition is to enter the 'Iron Man' world of the Triathlon – where you are likely to have to swim across a lake as well as run and cycle. Such is the popularity of this new sport that in the United States last year 1,000 competitions are said to have attracted 100,000 competitors; and Britain is rapidly following suit. Not all events are designed for Iron Men. In some the distances are quite modest: in June, for example, a weekend of events near Reading includes a family relay in which the three team members between them swim 200 yards, cycle five miles and run three miles (5). It is a new trend in sport, and a lot of people are starting to enjoy it, as well as making themselves a great deal fitter.

Walking

If you want to go walking with a group, you could join the Ramblers Association (6). They have 230 local rambling groups and are in touch with another 500 independent groups which organize walks, particularly at weekends. The walks are generally five to 12 miles – further than you are used to walking although you may well have been going at a faster pace. You should be able to achieve this distance without difficulty, but try to rest the day before your first walk. You could also think about consolidating the effort you have put in by arranging a walking holiday with other ramblers. (6)

More information

1 *Running.* Full itinerary of running events published in *Running* magazine.
2 *Fell running.* Membership of the Fell Runners Association costs £3 and provides a 100-race calendar of most of the year's events. Address: Norman Berry, 165 Penistone Road, Kirburton, Nr Huddersfield, Yorkshire.
3 *Orienteering.* List of all British events and entry details published in *Compass Sport* magazine, 37 Sandycombe Road, Twickenham, Middlesex. (Subcription £5.75).
4 *Cycling.* To help newcomers, *Cycling* magazine publishes a Club Finder column. A specialist cycle shop ought to provide information about local clubs. The British Cycling Federation, 116 Upper Woburn Place, London WC1, can provide a list of all racing and touring clubs.
5 *Triathlon.* Membership of the British Triathlon Association, £10, includes a list of all 1984 events. Address: Aleck Hunter, 3 Porters Avenue, Dagenham, Essex.
6 *Walking.* Membership of the Ramblers Association costs £6.50 per year, for which you receive a copy of their journal *Rucksack* four times a year and an annual guide to bed and breakfast places all over Britain. They also supply lists of path guides. Address: Ramblers Association, 1 Wandsworth Road, London SW8 2LJ. Ramblers Holidays Ltd (PO Box 43, Welwyn Garden City, Herts), who are associated with the Ramblers Association, organize walking holidays in a number of European countries as well as in Britain.

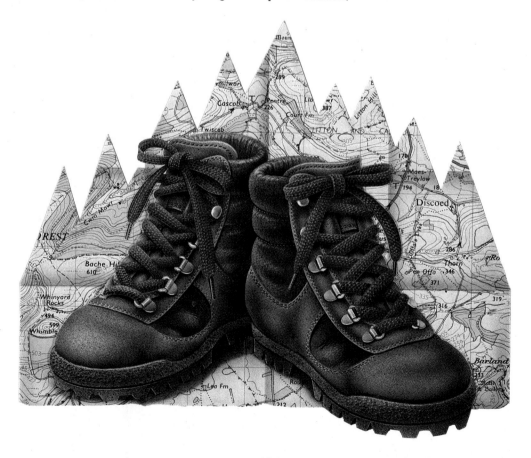

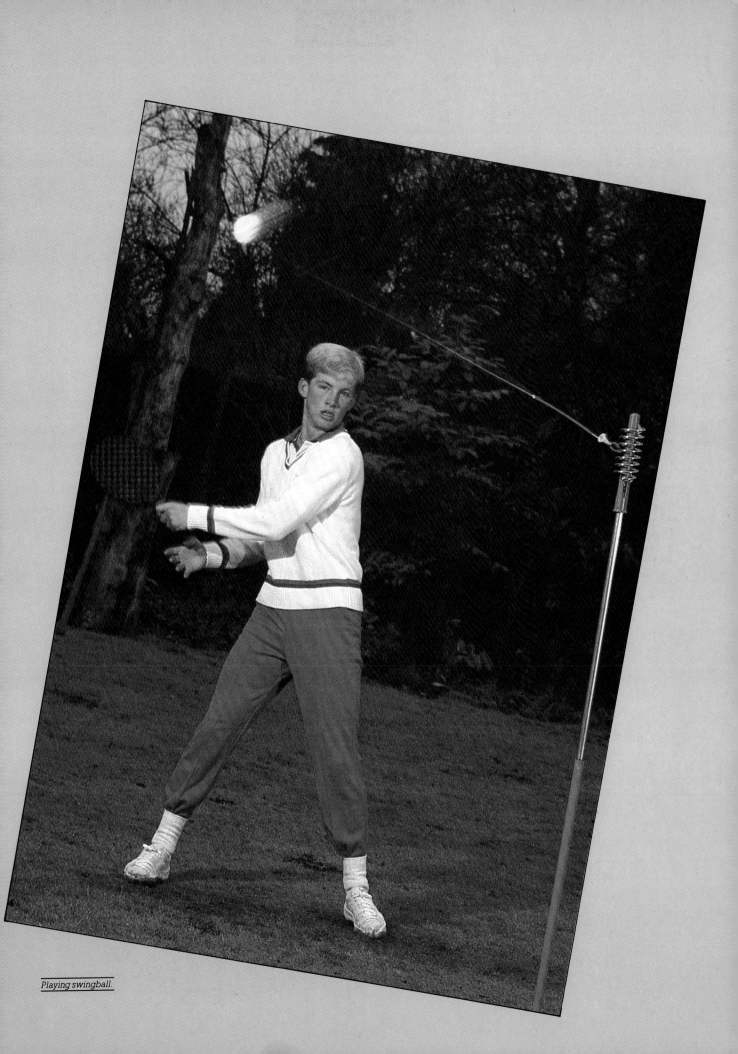

Playing swingball.

ACTIVITY

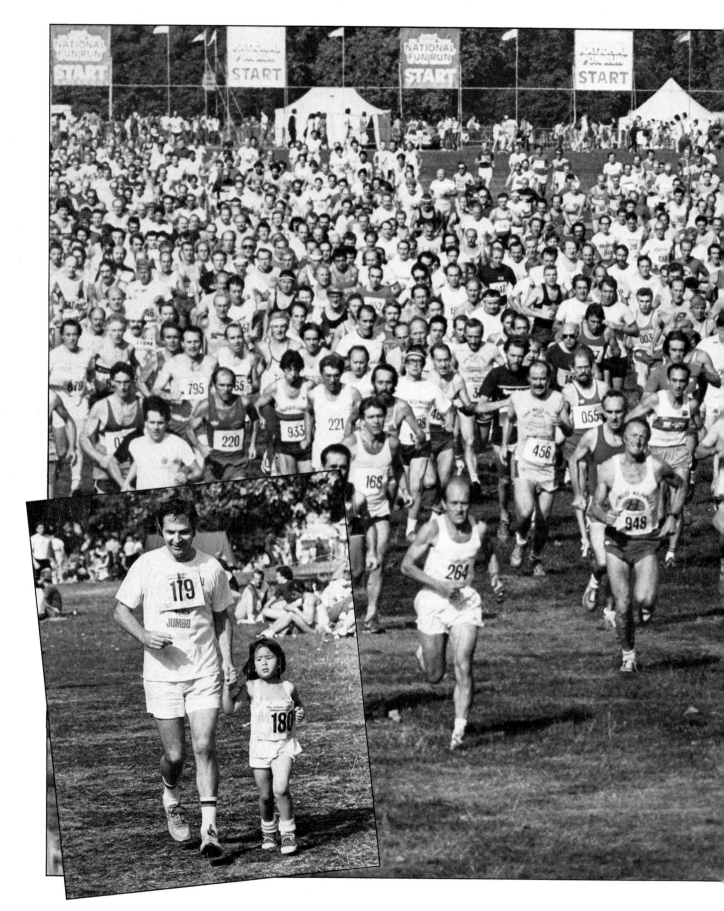

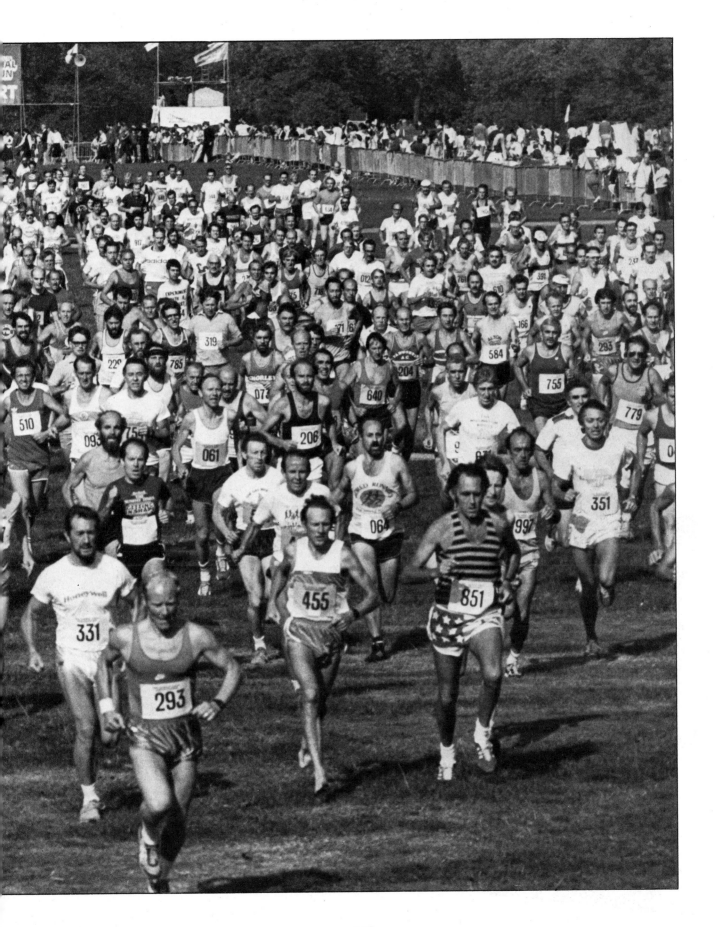

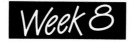
B FOR BEHAVIOUR

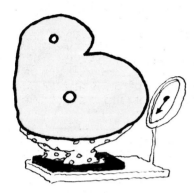

Nothing succeeds like success, the saying goes. But the approaching fulfilment of a goal may be a time of anxiety for many people. This is true whether the goal is, say, becoming the owner of your dream house, finishing a project in which you have invested a lot of energy, or slimming down to your ideal size. Any change of this kind, even when it's eagerly desired, is potentially stressful because it entails altering not only your behaviour but also your image of yourself. We grow comfortable with the image we have of ourselves and no matter how much we think we may want to change it, many of us hang on to an outdated idea of ourselves as if it were an old suit, fit for the jumble sale but still preferred to newer acquisitions because it is so reassuringly familiar.

Living with the New You

Not everyone will experience anxiety as they reach their desired shape, but some will. Women are more likely to suffer in this respect, firstly, because their sense of identity is more closely entwined with their body image, and when their bodies change a greater readjustment in self-image is involved; and, secondly, because they are more wary than men of success in general and find it harder to assimilate. Women are generally more motivated to achieve – whether status, wealth, slimness – out of a desire for approval and love than for the sake of the achievement itself, as a host of studies by social psychologists has shown.

Once success has been achieved women are more prone than men to fear that the very success they have longed for will alienate them from others. But success can also be a challenge, an exciting new departure, an assertion of freedom. Because change on the ABC Diet and Bodyplan is gradual and is based on a new lifestyle, you will naturally have been making the adjustments in self-image necessary for long-term success as you went along. Here are some other ways of preparing for and consolidating your success:

1. Challenge stereotypes of slimness that you may not know you are holding: Using your answers to the personal construct exercise last week, examine what expectations you have of slimness, both negative and positive. 'Most people who go on a diet feel that if they were thinner it would have profound consequences on their personal relationships', says Dr Hubert Lacey, senior lecturer in psychiatry at St. George's Hospital Medical School, London. If you are one of these people, you may be disappointed if you find, as you probably will, that relationships do not change very significantly at all. If they do alter markedly – because you are more self-confident – you must be able to handle the possible

consequences to prevent yourself from sabotaging your success. There is no reason, other than popular stereotypes and dubious reasoning, why being slim should equal being more sexy, or more powerful, or less able to to take care of yourself, or less caring, for instance. Slimness is what you make it. If you did not do last week's personal construct exercise, do it now, or just consider for a moment your own fantasy of what difference it will make to your life to be slim.

2. Have fun trying out new roles: Rehearse new ways of relating to people, of behaving, dressing, walking. Like an actor playing a part, immerse yourself in a different personality for a while. Choose one that isn't totally different from your own, suggests Dr Fay Fransella, who heads the Centre for Personal Construct Psychology in London and runs special groups for slimmers. Rehearse your new part mentally and try it out in practice. You don't have to believe you're that person, merely act *as if* you were. The point is to discover for yourself what happens if you think of yourself differently and behave in new ways, whether people will react differently to you or whether the world will seem changed. Try out more than one role if you like and find out what new behaviour you feel comfortable with. Don't make the mistake of waiting until some arbitrary goal is reached before allowing yourself to be more expressive with clothes and body language.

3. Strengthen your coping strategies: Come to see that you don't have to be upset even by upsetting events, that if you do get upset, it needn't last all day or drive you to food or drink or negative feelings about yourself. If anger is a problem try to become less fearful of expressing it and therefore more able to express it appropriately. Other psychological strategies for coping with unpleasant emotions include conceding that you may be wrong sometimes (a very threatening admission for some people); asserting your rights so that you do not feel victimized; and accepting that there are aspects of your personality that you do not care for but that these do not make you an unworthy person. Exercise will also give you a mental resilience to help you cope with change. The psychological methods you have learnt – relaxation, meditation, positive affirmations, guided imagery – can also help to pre-empt draining emotional upsets.

4. Keep track: Refusal to keep a record of your behaviour (food eaten, money spent, things achieved, as well as your body measurements) is a way of letting things slip until there's a crisis. Monitoring on a daily basis is an act of self-respect and a self-balancing process, a way of declaring that you're an adult and can manage. The people most successful at staying slim are those who get back on course as soon as they notice the fat creeping back. The least successful are those who gain it all back – and more – before tackling the problem. There's no need to be obsessive, but avoid escapism.

5. Be good to yourself: Many people find the idea of rewarding themselves very hard. It makes them feel uncomfortable or guilty. They're afraid of being boastful, of tempting fate, or of being selfish. Or they feel undeserving, although they may feel quite justified in spending large sums on others – their partners or children for example. Set small realistic goals and reward yourself with a treat as soon as you can after achieving a target. If you have a setback, don't be too hard on yourself. See yourself as having a problem amenable to change rather than as a failure.

6. Give your actions a wider meaning: If you exercise simply to get thinner, you may soon lose interest. When exercising becomes part of a whole network of associations to do with being fit, enjoying using your body, sharing the company of friends and so on, you greatly enhance your motivation. The same is true of food. If you eat pasta simply because it's recommended on the ABC Diet and Bodyplan it may lose its appeal after a few weeks. Be creative in using different shapes and colours of pasta, invent new ways to cook it and serve it at dinner parties. It will take on a whole new set of meanings and the richer the meanings attached to

any desired behaviour, the more established that behaviour becomes.

7. Take responsibility for your own life: To a certain extent we all need encouragement and structure to come from the outside. But for lasting success, the structure and motivation need to come from within. Build up as wide a network of support as possible until you feel ready to go it alone. Get together with health-conscious friends. Organize relaxation and exercise sessions at work, lobby for an office fridge to keep healthy food fresh, cajole the canteen into providing the sort of food you want. Above all create the kind of lifestyle you want around you, and be aware that you are making these changes for yourself. No-one else is responsible for your wellbeing.

8. Trust yourself: There are deliberately no precise quantities given in the guidelines on food in the Bodyplan because the idea is for you to get in touch with natural hunger as well as your body's other natural needs. Given the chance, your body works as a self-regulating mechanism. Listen to it. Trust it. It's the finest resource you have.

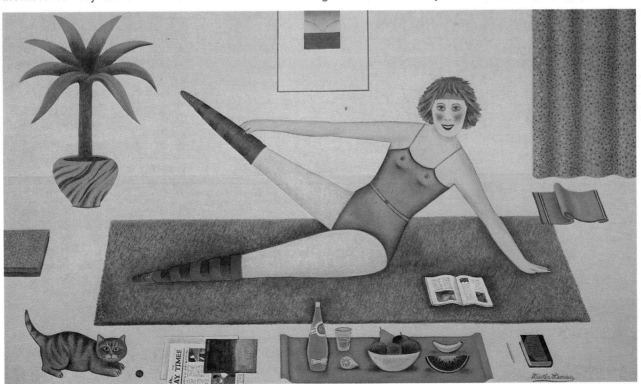

139

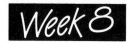

Week 8

C FOR CONSUMPTION

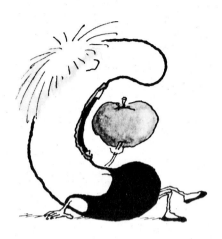

These are the principles of the Constant Energy Diet reduced to five DOs and five DONTs. Remind yourself of them in the weeks to come when you are thinking of what you should eat.

DOs

Eat 'slow food' such as pasta, rice and beans whenever you can.
Eat at least two apples a day.
Eat more vegetables and fruit (but not fruit juice).
Eat fish, chicken or turkey whenever you can rather than beef, lamb or pork.
Eat regular meals – at least three a day.
The Constant Energy Diet aims at balance, steering clear of the extremes of eating promoted by some slimming diets. Avoid these five common slimmers' errors:

DONTs

Don't consume a lot of sweet foods, particularly sweet drinks, which overload the system and lead to tiredness and hunger. They start a cycle of craving for more sweet food and will induce you to overeat.
Don't eat excessively fatty foods such as sausages, fried foods, biscuits, cakes or ice cream. Their fat content makes them high in calories and can lead to remorseless weight gain.
Don't attempt to slim by cutting down drastically on fats, because food is then digested too quickly and hunger returns again before the next meal time. Have butter with your baked potato, not cottage cheese.
Don't eat a high protein steak-and-lettuce type diet which causes a craving for carbohydrates and can lead to a self-defeating cycle of dieting and stuffing. Even lean steak is higher in fat and calories, weight for weight, than thick-cut chips or roast potatoes.
Don't rely on bran to conquer hunger. Too much bran can lead to a shortage of certain nutrients in the diet which may make slimming more difficult.

Entertaining

Entertaining is no problem with the Constant Energy Diet. There is no need for you to starve on cottage cheese and a lettuce leaf while guests tuck into rich fare made with lashings of cream and sugar. Everyone will enjoy these dishes and you will be able to stick to our dietary guidelines. The dishes succeed because of their subtle flavouring and choice of ingredients such as vegetables, grains, veal and fish, which are relatively low in fat. You can finish the meal with a deliciously tempting carrot cake carefully worked out to contain no more fat or sugar than necessary. The carrot cake also contains plenty of fibre so that it is filling – one slice should be quite enough. If you think the cake is more than you need at the end of the meal, serve fruit in the Greek style – cut up into pieces and arranged on a bed of chipped ice.

Recipes

Fish Mousse

This creamy fish mousse is, in fact, low in fat. It could be served as a first course for 6, or as a main course for 4 with a green salad. It can be made in advance and kept in the refrigerator overnight but will taste better if allowed to return to room temperature before being eaten.

12oz (350g) white fish, cod or haddock; 10fl oz (300ml) milk; bay leaf; 1 inch (2.5cm) piece of lemon peel; salt and pepper; 4oz (100-125g) French beans, cut in ½in pieces; 4oz (100-125g) carrots, cut in pieces 1in × ¼in sq.; 4oz (100-125g) smoked mackerel or salmon pieces; 4oz (100-125g) curd cheese; 1 tbsp lemon juice; 2 egg whites; 1 (0.4oz/11g) packet of gelatine. To decorate: Slices of cucumber; lemon slices; fresh herbs (dill is very good with the smoky flavour of the fish).

Poach the white fish in the milk with a bay leaf, lemon peel, salt and pepper until the fish is cooked (about 7 or 8 minutes). Remove the fish from the pan and when it is cool enough, remove and return the skin to the milk in the pan. Simmer gently to reduce the milk by one third. Strain into a jug and cool.
  Cook the prepared vegetables – the carrots first, then the beans – in 1 pint of barely salted water. Reserve the cooking liquid and lay the cooked vegetables on kitchen paper to drain and cool. Finely chop the smoked fish and mash it together with the cooked fish and the lemon juice.
  Put the curd cheese into a bowl and beat with a whisk, gradually adding 3fl oz (75ml) of the cooled milk until the mixture resembles thin cream. Heat 7fl oz (200ml) of the vegetable water in a pan. When hot, remove from the heat, sprinkle in the gelatine, stir to dissolve and allow to cool until tepid.
  Gradually fold the flaked fish into the curd cheese mixture then add the melted gelatine, mixing with a fork to incorporate as much air as possible. Put the bowl in the refrigerator to cool and whisk the egg whites until stiff. Fold them into the mousse. Ladle one third of the mousse into a 1½ pint (900ml) serving or soufflé dish, put in a

layer of half the vegetables and add another third of the fish, put in the rest of the vegetables and finish off with the rest of the fish. Smooth the top and decorate with slices of cucumber, lemon and fresh herbs. Leave 1 to 2 hours in the refrigerator to set.

Corn Chowder

This makes a admirable soup to start a meal. If you want to serve it as a main course you can add some fish. This is not then an authentic chowder, but the combination of the two is excellent.

2 rashers back bacon, cut in small pieces; 6oz (175g) shallots (or onions), sliced; 2 sticks celery, chopped; 12oz (350g) potatoes, cut in cubes; 12oz (350g) sweetcorn, off the cob, fresh or frozen; 1 pint (600ml) water; 1 pint (600ml) milk; salt and pepper; 1 tsp paprika; cream crackers or water biscuits

Cook the chopped bacon in a sauce pan until the fat runs, without browning. Add the chopped shallots or onions and celery, cover the pan and cook until transparent. Stir in the potato and add water. Simmer gently until the potatoes begin to soften. Add the milk and the sweetcorn and cook until the corn and potatoes are tender. Season with salt if necessary (salt added before the corn is cooked will toughen it), black pepper and a little paprika. To make a main course add 12oz (350g) of cooked scallops, crab, prawns or white fish, or a mixture of them all, and heat through before serving.

Serve in deep bowls. The crackers are crumbled into the chowder at the table.

Gazpacho

This cold Spanish soup is easy to prepare, requires no cooking, can be made ahead of time and will be all the better for a few hours in the fridge. It makes a good start to a summer meal.

2 slices stale white bread without crusts; 1 clove of garlic, crushed; 1 tbsp olive oil; 8oz (225g) ripe tomatoes, skinned and deseeded; 2 tbsp red wine vinegar; 4oz (100-125g) green pepper, chopped very finely; 4oz (100-125g) red pepper, chopped very finely; small bunch spring onions; 4 inch (10cm) chunk of cucumber, peeled and chopped very finely; parsley; 17fl oz (450ml) tomato juice; 10fl oz (300ml) chicken stock; salt and pepper

Soak the bread in water and squeeze dry. Put it in a large bowl with the crushed garlic, olive oil and tomatoes. Mash with a fork and add the vinegar. Chop the other vegetables and the parsley very finely and add them to the bowl. Stir in the tomato juice and the cold chicken stock, season and chill before serving. You can make the soup using a food processor and blender but it should not be processed for too long. It is much more interesting if the vegetables stay separate and a little crunchy.

Couscous

Couscous is made from hard durum wheat, like a rather course semolina. If it is unobtainable, the same aromatic stew could be served with rice. You will need a suitable pan and close fitting steamer, and a piece of butter muslin or clean cotton fabric.

12oz (350g) couscous; 2lb (1kg) chicken, cut into joints, or chicken pieces with the bone in; 6oz (175g) onion, sliced; 8oz (225g) carrots, sliced; 1lb (450g) tomatoes or an 8oz (225g) tin tomatoes; 8oz (225g) courgettes, sliced and salted; 4oz (110-125g) dried chick peas, soaked and pre-cooked, or 10oz (300g) tin of chick peas; 2tbsp olive or sunflower oil; 1tsp ginger or 1 inch (2.5cm) piece of fresh ginger, grated; 1tsp cinnamon; 1tsp ground cumin; 10fl oz (300ml) chicken stock; salt and pepper; small knob of butter. For the Sauce: 1 small tin of harissa (hot sauce, available from ethnic food shops). Or 1½tbsp tomato paste; 1 clove garlic, crushed; ½tsp ground coriander; 1 to 2 tsp chilli powder, all mixed together.

Soak the couscous in a bowl with enough water to just cover it (about 15fl oz or 400ml). Mix the grains around with your hands to make sure there are no lumps. Heat the oil in a round fireproof casserole or heavy saucepan and cook the onions until transparent, stir in the carrots and cook for a moment or two before adding the chicken. Let the chicken brown on all sides then stir in the spices, which should cook for a few minutes before the tomatoes and stock are added.

Let the casserole simmer while you transfer the soaked couscous into a steamer lined with a piece of muslin. Fold the muslin over the couscous and do not put a lid on the steamer. Put the steamer over the pan, plugging any gaps round the edge with a small piece of aluminium foil. After 30 minutes' cooking, transfer the couscous to a bowl and add a little water to it before stirring it again with a fork to eliminate any lumps. Add the courgettes and chick peas to the pan, add a pinch of salt, return the couscous to the steamer and cook for a further 30 minutes. At the end of an hour the stew should be ready to serve. Moisten the harissa or the home-made sauce with 2 or 3 tablespoons of the gravy from the casserole.

To serve, put the couscous into a heated serving dish with a small lump of butter and give each person a portion of this with some of the stew. Let them help themselves to the hot sauce. I serve a bowl of yoghurt with this dish which people can help themselves to if they burn their mouths; it is far better than water for soothing the mouth.

Veal in a Loaf

This is an easy casserole which can be put in the oven to cook while you are busy. Assemble it at the last minute and serve with a bowl of salad.

1¼lb (550g) stewing veal; 6oz (175g) onion, sliced; 6oz (175g) carrots, sliced; 6oz (175g) mushrooms, cut in half; 1 clove garlic; 2fl oz (50ml) white wine; 15fl oz (400ml) chicken stock; 2tbs olive or sunflower oil; salt and pepper; 1 bay leaf; 1 tbs paprika; 1 small carton of yoghurt; 1 dsp cornflour; medium sized loaf of brown or white bread

Preheat the oven to 350°F (180°C, gas mark 4). Slice the top off the loaf of bread, scoop out the middle. Put the hollow loaf and the lid into the oven to crisp up for 20 minutes while you prepare the casserole.

Put the oil in a heavy casserole and sauté the sliced onions and the carrots until just beginning to brown. Remove them from the pan and brown the veal, trimmed and cut into 1 inch (2.5cm) squares. Cook a few pieces at a time. When all the veal is brown, add the crushed garlic and the paprika and stir over a gentle heat for a moment or two. Add the wine and let it simmer, scraping up any residue from the bottom of the pan. Return the onions and carrots to the casserole and add a little salt, some black pepper and the bay leaf. Pour on the warmed stock and put the casserole in a low oven, 300°F (150°C, gas mark 2), for two hours. Add the cleaned, halved mushrooms to the casserole half an hour before the end of the cooking time.

When the veal is tender, take the casserole from the oven and put it over a low heat. Mix the cornflour and a little water and stir into the yoghurt, in a bowl. Ladle a spoonful or two of the juice from the casserole and stir together gently. Pour the mixture carefully into the casserole and stir gently until the juices thicken. Stir only in one direction or the yoghurt may curdle. Simmer a moment or two longer then pour into the loaf case and serve with a piece of the toasty bread.

Carrot Cake

This is a very moist cake, rather like a good gingerbread. It can be eaten warm as a pudding or served as a cake. The quantity should be enough for 6 to 8 people.

2oz (50g) soft light brown sugar; 6oz (175g) apple and pear spread (available from health food stores); 4oz (110-125g) butter; 6oz (175g) grated carrot; 2oz (50g) dried apricots, chopped; 2oz (50g) raisins; 8fl oz (225ml) water; 8oz (225g) plain white flour, or a mixture of plain and wholemeal; 2tsp ginger; 4oz (110-125g) ground almonds; 2tsp bicarbonate of soda.

Grease a 9in (22.5cm) cake tin and line the bottom with baking parchment or greaseproof paper. Put the butter, sugar, apple and pear spread, carrot, apricots, raisins and water into the saucepan and melt together slowly. Stir until mixed then bring to the boil and simmer briskly for 5 minutes. Leave until nearly cold.

Sift the dry ingredients into a bowl and add the mixture from the saucepan. Stir thoroughly but quickly and pour quickly into the prepared tin. Cook in a pre-heated oven at 350°F (180°C, gas mark 4) for approximately 1 hour. Test with a skewer to make sure it is done. If the cake appears to be burning on top put a piece of greaseproof paper loosely over the top for the last 15 minutes of cooking time. Cool in the tin for 15 minutes and then turn out on to a rack and peel the paper off the bottom of the cake.

CONSUMPTION

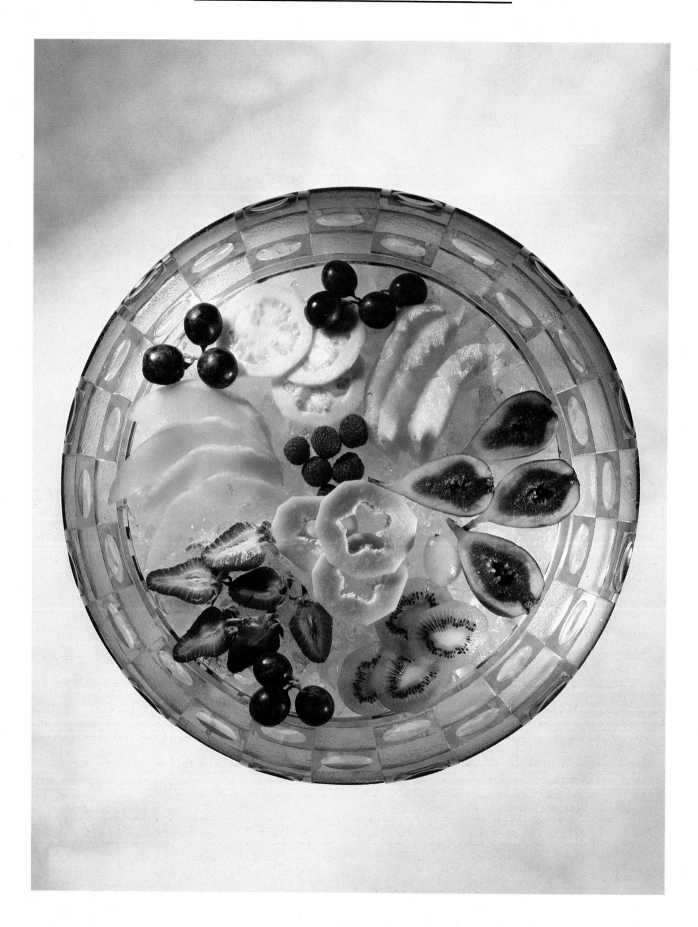

Fruit on Ice

Choose from: pineapple; mango; melon; pawpaw; grapes; peaches; figs; cherries; apricots; raspberries; watermelon; plums; oranges; tangerines; lychees; red currants; ripe gooseberries.

Buy fruit in season, making sure it is ripe and sweet enough to eat without sugar.

Take the contents of 3 or 4 icetrays, wrap the cubes in a strong, clean tea towel and crush the ice with a mallet or rolling pin. Put the crushed ice in a polythene bag and store in the freezer.

Wash and prepare the fruit, cutting up the larger fruits into smaller portions and dividing the grapes or currants into small bunches. Cover the fruit with cling film and chill until required.

Put the crushed ice in a large dish or bowl and arrange the fruit on it. Decorate.

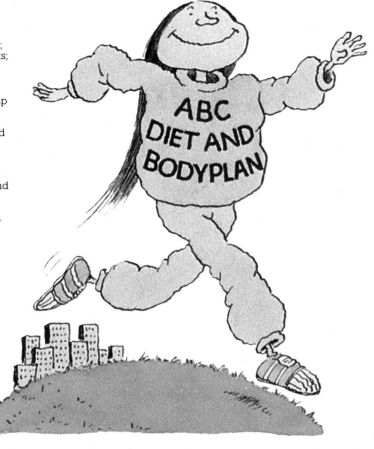

YOUR ABC DIARY: Week Eight					Starting date:			
	WALKING		JOGGING/ WALKING		SWIMMING		HOME WORKOUT	OTHER EXERCISE (e.g. cycling)
	Mins	Miles*	Mins	Miles*	Mins	Lengths	Mins	Mins
Monday								
Tuesday								
Wednesday								
Thursday								
Friday								
Saturday								
Sunday								
TOTAL								

* approximate distance, optional

ABC ROAD TEST	mins		mph		SWIMMING TIME TEST	lengths	mins

BODY MEASUREMENTS	Date / /	Chest	Waist	Hips	Arms	Legs	Weight

THE AUTHORS

Oliver Gillie is medical correspondent of *The Sunday Times*. He has been commended three times in National Press Awards and has won several other awards for scientific and medical writing. He is the author of "The Living Cell," "How To Stop Smoking," "Who Do You Think You Are?", "The Sunday Times Guide To The World's Best Food" (co-author) and "The Sunday Times Book Of Body Maintenance" (co-author).

Susana Raby is a journalist specialising in medicine and psychology. She holds an MA in modern languages (Oxon) and a BSc in psychology (London).

Illustrations Credits
Abril-Zefa 101   David Bailey 18, 34, 50, 66, 82, 98, 114, 130   Mike Brett 133   Camera Press 38, 39, 54, 76, 103   Femina 29
Finbar Tinto 57   Colin Frewin 15, 23, 25, 37, 87, 102   Grizelda Holderness 107   Grundy + Northedge 29   Brad Holland 91
Robert Jones 21   Peter Knapp 22   Kobal Collection 44, 73, 120, 129   Anita Kunz 2, 43   Martin Leman 139   Allan Manham 27
James Merrell 74, 86   Chris Nash 40   National Gallery, London 104   Graham Percy 123   Roger Perry 53, 116, 119
Picturepoint 106   Ian Pollock 31   David Reed 41, 59, 135   Arthur Robins 10, 12, 13, 14, 20, 21, 26 ,28, 36, 42, 46, 52, 56, 58, 68,
76, 80, 84,.90, 94, 100, 104, 110, 116, 122, 124, 126, 132, 138, 140, 143   Tony Stone Photo Library Worldwide 55, 69, 118
Sunday Times 136   Mario Testino 6, 7, 63, 85, 102   Topham 5, 24, 88, 93, 105, 109, 125   Tessa Traeger 30, 49, 62, 95, 111,
127, 142   Claus Wickrath 79   Harry Willock 47, 61, 134   Philip Wilson 11, 71